DIABETES

A practical new guide to healthy living

James W. Anderson, MD

Arco Publishing, Inc.
New York

To Gay, Kathy and Steve with love

Published 1981 by Arco Publishing, Inc.
219 Park Avenue South, New York, N.Y. 10003

© James W. Anderson, MD 1981

First published in the United Kingdom
in 1981 by Martin Dunitz Limited, London

Library of Congress Cataloging in Publication Data
Anderson, James (James Wingo), 1936–
  Diabetes, a practical new guide to healthy living.
  Includes index.
  1. Diabetes. I. Title.
RC660.A62   616.4′62   81-66801
ISBN 0-668-05328-3   AACR2

Jacket photograph by John Clutterbuck

Printed in the United States of America

Dr James W. Anderson is Professor of Medicine and Clinical Nutrition at the University of Kentucky in Lexington. For the past twenty years he has specialized in the treatment of diabetes as well as maintaining a busy medical practice. His research team at the University of Kentucky has developed and tested the new high carbohydrate and fiber (HCF) diets which help diabetic patients to control their condition. Currently Dr Anderson directs the Diabetes Service at the Veterans Administration Medical Center where he has an active research and teaching program.

He is married and the father of two children. The Anderson family enjoy travelling together. Dr Anderson believes in regular excercise, which he takes by jogging and playing tennis. He also collects stamps.

CONTENTS

INTRODUCTION

In the last decade many exciting new breakthroughs have developed in the treatment of diabetes. Researchers have identified certain viruses that can cause diabetes in children. Special research tests can now be used to identify children who are likely to develop diabetes. Some diabetic patients have been cured with pancreas transplants; others have been brought into excellent control with an artificial pancreas. The dreaded complications of diabetes such as blindness, kidney failure and gangrene have been feared far more than the disease itself. Recent evidence indicates that many of these problems can be avoided altogether, or at least greatly diminished in frequency, by excellent diabetic control. To me, the most exciting challenge is to translate these dazzling scientific developments into practical measures that can be used by the diabetic to improve his or her day-to-day well-being.

Many scientific experiments with humans and with animals have shown that diabetic complications such as eye and kidney problems are related to abnormally high blood sugars. For example, dogs which are made diabetic by removing their pancreas develop the eye and kidney problems seen in some human diabetics. These dogs' problems can be prevented by vigorous treatment with insulin to maintain excellent blood sugar levels. If you are diabetic, learning to control your blood sugar is your best insurance for the future.

We now have the tools available to provide good diabetic control for most patients. I will be explaining in this book how you can use these tools. First, we know that while a consistent diet is important for everyone, it is vital for diabetics. At my hospital we have developed a new diet program which smooths out swings in blood sugar and reduces insulin needs; most diabetic patients find these diets appetizing and practical. Second, we now have an excellent choice of insulins available. The purified pork insulin may be as effective as human insulin; and much better information is now available about how to inject insulin. Third, we realize the importance of exercise in lowering the blood sugar and promoting good general health. Fourth, for you to reap the greatest benefit, it is vitally important for the whole health-care team to teach you how to take care of your diabetes in your daily life. Finally, better equipment and techniques are now available to monitor your blood sugar level. Laboratory tests can be used that will give a good estimate of your blood sugar during the previous six weeks since your last visit to the doctor. Also, more patients have started to measure their own blood sugar using home monitors. To take advantage of these improved methods of controlling your blood sugar you should try to learn as much as you can about your diabetes. You cannot expect to master your diabetes if you don't know what to look for and why you are looking for it. Knowledge of your diabetes is the key to better control.

Taking care of your diabetes is like being captain of an American football team. In American football, when your team has the ball, you the captain must decide whether to run, throw or kick the ball. You need always to anticipate what the other team is going to do. If you do get into trouble, you can ask for help from your coaches. You can play the game much better once you know a great deal about football, how the players in your team work together and what the other team is likely to do.

You must be in control of your diabetes like the captain of a football team. You will need to decide what to eat, how much exercise to take and perhaps also, about adjusting your insulin dose. You will be able to take better care of your diabetes once you know more about it – how diabetes functions and the possible problems you might face as a result. The more you can anticipate problems, the better you will be at controlling your diabetes. If you do get into trouble, you need to call your coaches – doctors, nurses or dietitians – for help. I have written this book to help you be a better captain of your diabetes.

Being the captain isn't easy as you cannot blame someone else for your own mistakes. In fact, it would be much easier to do everything only under your doctor's instructions. The problem with this is that you have to live with your diabetes twenty-four hours a day, seven days a week. You may have to make decisions on the spot when your doctor may not be around. Your doctor might have many diabetic patients and if you call him at home, say at 7.00 am, he may not remember all the details of your case, however interested he is. So you must know more about your diabetes than anyone else to enable you to make decisions.

When you do call your doctor bring him up to date on your situation by telling him: what your problem is; how much insulin you are taking and at what time of day; then diplomatically tell him what you had considered doing. Your doctor may well make a different suggestion but he will want to know how you had planned to handle the situation. This will give him an idea of how well you are coping with your diabetes.

To ensure success, you and your doctor need to work together as a team. Your doctor has had many years of training and experience, treating many different types of diabetic problems. He will be directing your general course of action but you are the one with the responsibility for day-to-day control of your own diabetes. Good two-way communications between you and your doctor are essential.

I have written this book in response to the hundreds of requests from patients, nurses, dietitians and others. This is the first time that the high-fiber diets we have developed specially for diabetics at Lexington, Kentucky, have ever been published for a wide readership apart from in medical and scientific journals. These diets have already attracted wide interest in the United States and led to dramatic improvements for many of our patients.

Inevitably in a book like this there just isn't sufficient space to write in depth about every facet of diabetes. I have attempted to deal with all the important features but inevitably some diabetics will want to find out more about particular aspects. Also, some people want to know about their diabetes in more detail than others. What I have tried to provide is a general introduction to the nature of diabetes, including the most important ways to control your blood sugar and avoid complications; practical suggestions for coping in your everyday life; and guidelines for planning your own high-fiber diet. And to help readers from other countries when they read the book, alternatives have been included in some places where the terminology or medical practice may vary slightly.

I firmly believe that being diabetic today need not be as great a burden as it once was. I have no doubt not only that facing up to your diabetes and taking the steps I suggest in this book will help you to control your diabetes and lead a full and rewarding life, but also that taking regular exercise and having a sensible diet will improve your total health and reduce your risk of having a heart attack and other possible complications.

If I am able to help you and perhaps also your family cope better with your diabetes by creating better understanding then I will feel that this book has achieved its purpose.

Please note

Some aspects of the treatment of diabetes vary from region to region and country to country. For example, different types of insulin and syringes are used in different countries. But significant variations have been incorporated in this book wherever possible. However, you and your doctor will need to work out your own program. You should not change your diet, nor, if you are taking insulin or pills, change your dose, under any circumstances without checking with your doctor.

1 WHAT IS DIABETES AND WHAT CAUSES IT?

To be in control of your diabetes you first need to understand it. If you are diabetic your body is unable to break down and use your foods properly. Excessive amounts of sugar, instead of being burned up as energy, accumulate in the blood and spill over into the urine. Too much fat, usually derived from fatty food such as butter, cheese and fried foods, also builds up in the blood instead of being used by your body. Protein from meat, fish and poultry is converted into sugar instead of producing muscles and replacing damaged tissues. Over a period of time this high level of sugar in the blood can damage the eyes, kidneys, nerves and other parts of the body.

All these problems are due to one basic cause – the diabetic's inability to produce enough insulin to use these foods properly. The following example, from my experience, conveys the early dilemma of the diabetic. The questions raised are typical of those asked by the thousands of new diabetics each year.

Recently Elizabeth, a forty-nine year-old woman, came to me to find out if she had diabetes. As she knew her father was diabetic she had a blood test, which showed that her blood sugar was high. She had many questions which built up to an almost explosive point. Did she have diabetes? Would it go away? Would she have to take insulin shots? Could she still work? How long would she live? Would it affect her sight? What about gangrene . . .? I tried to calm her down until we had more information.

Blood tests told us that Elizabeth did indeed have diabetes, so our team started explaining to her more about the disease. She is what is known as an adult-type diabetic who usually does not require insulin injections. A minority of diabetics have the juvenile-type and they usually do need insulin. I will be explaining more about the important difference between them later in this chapter. A nurse taught her how to test her urine. A dietitian instructed her about our special kind of high-fiber diet. We all talked with her, answered her questions, and gave her printed information to take home and read. Over the next few months Elizabeth learned a great deal about diabetes. Fortunately, in her case we have been able to control it and she has not needed insulin injections or pills. But for many people the disease takes a more severe course. So in this chapter I will try to answer some of the questions generally asked by a new diabetic.

What causes diabetes?

Diabetes may result from several different causes. In non-diabetics, the pancreas, a large gland close to the stomach, has special cells called beta-cells. These produce insulin – a chemical messenger known as a hormone. Insulin is needed to regulate the use of sugar in the blood which the body uses for energy.

If someone's entire pancreas has been removed or seriously damaged for any reason, diabetes will develop as insulin is not made. For example, drinking excessive amounts of alcohol for many years can destroy the pancreas and produce diabetes. In India and certain other parts of the world, a pancreas-destroying infection is a common cause.

Certain diseases, too, are accompanied by large amounts of hormones or substances that fight the effects of insulin in the body. If the pituitary, thyroid, or adrenal glands are producing large quantities of their hormones, temporary diabetes may develop. Once the basic gland problems have been corrected, and insulin can again work unopposed, the diabetes disappears.

Most cases of diabetes are caused because the beta-cells are damaged by an unknown process. The tendency to develop the condition is usually inherited, and in these cases the cells starts to die slowly from the time of birth. With luck though, beta-cells may make enough insulin to prevent the development of diabetes for 70 or 80 years. In fact, only a quarter of all diabetics develop their condition before the age of fifty, and about half of all cases develop it between the ages of fifty and sixty-five. A major puzzle is why diabetes affects some children but spares most potential diabetics until they have reached middle age.

In some children infection of the pancreas by a virus such as mumps or flu may be responsible for diabetes. In one small American town, a very serious outbreak of mumps was followed by an epidemic of diabetes in children. Over a three-month period in this town far more children developed diabetes than doctors would normally have expected. The link between a virus infection and diabetes is therefore very strong.

One child for example, developed a viral infection and subsequently died with severe diabetes. On post-mortem a virus was identified in the beta-cells of his pancreas. This virus was extracted from the pancreas and injected into mice who developed diabetes, and the same virus was found in their beta-cells as well. At the present time, we do not know how often a viral infection is responsible for diabetes in children. Most experts think that viruses only cause diabetes in children who already have a tendency towards the disease.

In most adults, the cause of diabetes appears to be related to the beta-cells running out of insulin. In some ways, running out of insulin is like your car running out of gas. Some people drive sensibly, never speed and can travel many miles on a tank of gas. Others are always making a fast start, racing the engine, speeding up, then braking sharply and driving too fast; they may get less than half the mileage from a tank of gas compared to the sensible driver. The best way to combat a tendency to develop diabetes is to eat sensibly. Overeating and carrying too much weight wastes insulin. Staying slim and eating the kind of foods described in chapters eight and nine seems to slow down the gradual slide into a diabetic state.

Who is most likely to develop diabetes?

Diabetes occurs more commonly among overweight people, women, the elderly, and the poor. I will be talking about the staggering association between diabetes and obesity later in the book. Diabetes is almost 50 per cent more common among women than men, about three women develop it for every two men. The reasons for these differences are still unclear. Pregnancies may contribute to the unmasking of diabetes, as women who have many children (over 12) are much more likely to develop it than women who have never had children. Also, as women on average live longer than men they have a greater chance of developing diabetes, as there are more older women than men.

With each additional ten years of age, the risk of developing diabetes increases. Among people over sixty-five years old, diabetes is 60 times more common than in persons under seventeen, and individuals are 20 times more likely to develop it during their seventieth year of life than during their fifteenth year.

In Western countries, diabetes is more common among the poor than more affluent groups. In the United States in 1973, for example, the number of people with diabetes was three times greater when the family income was less than $5000 per year than when it exceeded $10 000. Many other factors, such as race, diet, environment, and physical activity, influence the risk of developing the disease – for instance, American Indians (particularly the Pimas) have very high rates of diabetes, possibly due to their obesity, inactivity and diet, whereas the people of Bangladesh have very low rates.

What does insulin do?

Insulin made by the pancreas acts as a catalyst for the passage of a simple sugar called glucose through the blood stream into the muscle and fat cells. It acts rather like a key with the cell wall having a 'padlock' called an insulin receptor. When insulin, the key, fits into the lock, the receptor (the cell wall) opens to allow more sugar to enter. Insulin also speeds up the use of sugar in the cell, by directly stimulating the burning of sugar as fuel and its storage in the body. Fat storage is also helped by insulin, as well as the manufacture of protein in the muscles. So, insulin directs the energy storage program of the body and enhances the muscle-building process.

In non-diabetics the level of sugar in their blood, known as blood sugar, is kept within a fairly narrow range. Even after a very large meal containing a large amount of sugar, the blood sugar doesn't usually rise above 150 mg per 100 ml (8 mmol per liter). Blood sugar is mainly regulated by the insulin released by the beta-cells of the pancreas; as the blood sugar rises, more insulin is released, and when it falls the pancreas stops putting out insulin. In non-diabetics enough insulin is produced to control the blood sugar, rather similar to the way a central heating thermostat controls room temperature.

What happens as diabetes develops?

The pancreas can be compared to a car battery, with insulin as the spark the battery produces to ignite the car's gas. Without insulin the body is unable to burn up the energy it needs. If your car battery goes dead you'll need a boost from another battery to get your car started. Similarly, if your pancreas goes dead or isn't able to produce enough insulin then you need a boost of insulin from another source.

As diabetes develops, the ability of the pancreas to release insulin declines. After each meal the blood sugar slowly creeps higher and higher. Measurement of blood sugar before breakfast, the first meal of the day after getting up in the morning, is known as the fasting blood sugar level. Very soon even this is elevated. When a lean person gets to the stage where his or her blood sugar is abnormally high before breakfast, the insulin level in the pancreas is usually quite low (see diagram). When the fasting blood sugar is above 200 mg per 100 ml (11 mmol per liter), and when the blood sugar climbs above 300 mg per 100 ml (17 mmol per liter) after meals, most people have symptoms of diabetes.

Do I have diabetes?

As diabetes develops over many years in adults, it is often difficult to tell

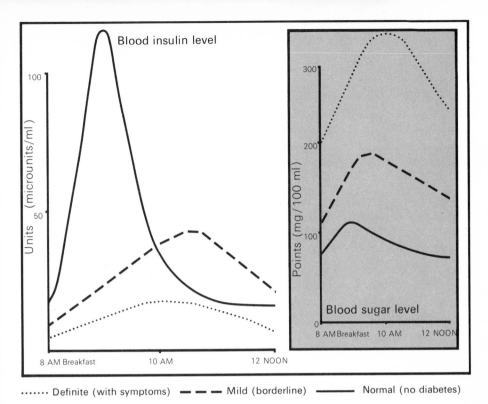

······ Definite (with symptoms)　━ ━ ━ Mild (borderline)　━━━━ Normal (no diabetes)

LEFT: Within about an hour after eating breakfast the definite diabetic's blood insulin does not rise sufficiently to cope with the glucose eaten.
RIGHT: His blood sugar, though, rises sharply.
　The non-diabetic's blood insulin rises sharply after breakfast to cope with the additional glucose. The balancing of insulin to glucose keeps the blood sugar down naturally in the non-diabetic.

when somebody crosses the border from being non-diabetic to diabetic. For every ten recognized diabetics there are at least five more unrecognized, or 'borderline diabetics'.

　Most experts agree that when the fasting blood sugar level is more than 130 mg per 100 ml (7 mmol per liter) on two separate occasions, a definite diagnosis of diabetes can be made. If the fasting blood sugar is below 100 mg per 100 ml ($5\frac{1}{2}$ mmol per liter) there is no diabetes. Borderline cases have fasting blood glucose values between 100 and 130 mg per 100 ml ($5\frac{1}{2}$ and 7 mmol per liter).

Is diabetes inherited?

This is a question my patients often ask me. Young couples who plan to have children are naturally very concerned about this point, especially if there is a history of diabetes in either partner's family.

13

The answer is that virtually every case of diabetes is inherited. Many experts think that in the United States, for example, almost one person in four has the genetic tendency to develop diabetes, and will develop it if they are exposed to certain viruses, or become overweight, or have other stresses to the pancreas.

Diabetes can include several different diseases which all produce a high blood sugar. In addition to the inherited defects of the beta-cells, diabetes can also be caused by either severe infections of the pancreas, surgical removal of the pancreas or other processes which can damage beta-cells.

Because at the moment we cannot determine the exact cause of diabetes in most people, it is impossible to predict how likely their relatives are to develop the disease. So the inheritance pattern of one form of diabetes may be different from other types. From my experience, I think that diabetes tends to follow this pattern: if both parents have diabetes, all their children will have the tendency to develop diabetes; some may develop the juvenile-type, others may not develop diabetes until middle age and some children may never develop it at all. The *tendency*, however, is still there.

In identical twins, if one has diabetes there is a very high likelihood that the other will eventually develop it. In fact scientists have found that for any sets of identical twins, if either twin develops adult-type diabetes there is a 100 per cent likelihood that the other will eventually develop it as well. If, however, either identical twin should develop juvenile-type diabetes the chances of the other twin becoming diabetic are 50 per cent.

In general, if one member of the family has diabetes, the chances of other members of the immediate family (father, mother, brothers or sisters) developing it are about five times greater than in a family with no predisposition to the disease.

Types of diabetes

Juvenile

These type of diabetics have virtually no ability to make insulin themselves. This form is also known as insulin-dependent diabetes mellitus. Without insulin reserves these individuals are vulnerable to ketosis, a condition resulting from an accumulation of fat by-products called ketones in the blood. This condition is described in more detail later in this chapter. When plenty of insulin is available very few ketones are made but when fat is burned without insulin being available a lot of fat gets converted into ketones. A build-up of these acidic by-products cause acidosis and ketoacidosis which can lead to coma. Virtually all diabetic children and a very small percentage of diabetic adults have this type.

In juvenile-type diabetes, boys and girls are equally prone, and instead of obesity being an important contributory factor most juvenile-type diabetics are lean. Diabetes among children and teenagers is often triggered by a childhood infection such as a virus. For a time, the virus may mask the diabetes as the parents associate their child's symptoms with the fever. The first appearance of diabetes often seems sudden and dramatic. Also, all children's blood-sugar levels fluctuate much more widely than an adult's due to their greater physical activity and the needs of children's growth. The following are some of the main clues for detecting diabetes in children.

Symptoms of the juvenile-type

Urination   Often the earliest clue to diabetes is an increase in the amount of urine passed. Bed-wetting sometimes leads to the first suspicions that the child might be diabetic.

Thirst   To keep up with the loss of urine, diabetics drink more fluids. If the child has lots of Koolaid®, orange juice, lemonade or cola drinks the extra sugar in these drinks may accelerate the development of obvious diabetes.

Weight loss   Diabetic children usually lose, or fail to gain, weight until they are treated.

Unsatisfied hunger   This may occur even though the child is eating plenty of food. Once again, candies, cookies, cakes and other sweet foods may make the diabetes worse.

Cessation of growth   Usually children get taller and gain weight in a predictable way until their mid-teens. The development of diabetes may hold back growth in height until insulin therapy has started; then diabetic children catch up and resume their normal growth pattern.

Irritability   This can be a very early sign of diabetes. As many things affect the emotions of children, parents may not readily notice a change in their behaviour. If a happy, contented baby suddenly becomes much more fussy and also needs to have his diapers or nappies changed more frequently you should consider diabetes as a possible cause.

Drowsiness or coma   These are late stages in the development of diabetes. Usually we see children before they get to this stage. However, some type of illness (such as the flu, diarrhea or pneumonia) may quickly bring on a state of coma. The earliest clues to ketoacidosis and coma may be rapid breathing, nausea, sleepiness, and then coma (when the child can't easily be awakened).

Adult

85 per cent of all diabetics have the adult-type and retain some capacity to produce insulin themselves. Often this type of diabetic's pancreas produces a partial supply of insulin which the body is not able to utilize properly. Also in many cases of adult-type diabetes there is a tendency to be overweight, and the person's extra fat cells create an extra strain for their pancreas which is unable to produce enough insulin.

Although some adult-type diabetics do need insulin injections or antidiabetes pills, known as oral hypoglycemic pills, most of them can keep their diabetes under control by diet alone. For this reason this type is sometimes known as non-insulin dependent diabetes mellitus. Most people with this tendency do not develop the disease until they are at least thirty-five years old and many are well into middle age. They rarely have ketoacidosis and only go into coma if they become dehydrated (caused by a great loss of body fluids), and develop very high blood sugars.

Symptoms of the adult-type

Fatigue   The earliest clue to diabetes in adults is a vague feeling that things are not quite right. If you are developing diabetes you may notice a lack of energy, you feel tired much more easily, you find yourself thinking more sluggishly than usual, and there is fogginess of memory.

Urination at night   Most adults sleep through the night without getting up to pass urine. The need to urinate once or more may be an early clue to diabetes.

Constant thirst   If you produce a lot of urine you will need to drink more fluids to replace that water you lose. Some people have to drink water or other fluids every 15 to 30 minutes as they develop diabetes.

Weight loss   Although adult-type diabetics are usually overweight they sometimes seem to lose a little weight before they are first treated by a doctor.

What makes the diabetic's blood sugar go up?

When the blood sugar is too high sugar spills over into the urine. The kidney acts like a wooden dam built across a creek to form a small lake. With heavy rains the water level rises above the dam and water floods the downstream area. When the blood sugar goes above a level of about 180 mg per 100 ml (10 mmol per liter) the kidneys are unable to hold the sugar back and it floods into the urine. As long as the blood sugar is below the 160 mg per 100 ml to 200 mg per 100 ml level (9 to 11 mmol per liter), sugar is not spilled into the urine.

You can see from the diagram that as diabetes develops both the blood sugar and the urine sugar climb higher and higher. To keep all this sugar constantly dissolved in water the kidneys make more and more urine. The thirst centers of the body tell you to drink more water. So, in the early stages of the disease there is both excessive thirst and urination. The symptoms mentioned before – increased urination and weight loss as well as weakness and tiredness – are also direct results of the high blood sugar. This is followed by drowsiness, lethargy and the juvenile-type coma.

If diabetes is allowed to continue unchecked over a long period the following can develop due to the build-up of blood sugars.

Blurred vision   Sometimes patients are referred to me by their eye doctor after complaining of blurred vision. They find when they look up from reading a newspaper and try to see someone across the room that their vision suddenly becomes blurred. This fuzzy vision is caused by the accumulation of sugar and sugar products in the lens of the eye (see diagram page 81). The high blood sugars cause excessive sugar to pour into the lens and other tissues. This is then converted into various sugar products which the body is unable to burn up properly. These sugar products draw more water into the lens until it swells.

When the lens is swollen it takes longer to change the focus from near to distant vision. Fortunately, these abnormalities can be completely corrected by restoring the blood sugar to normal, and the lens slowly recovers in four to six weeks. If you wear glasses you should not get a new prescription for your lenses until six weeks after your blood sugar has been stabilized.

Skin infections   Poorly controlled diabetics are more likely to get pimples, boils and carbuncles. This tendency is entirely due to high blood sugars, and can be completely reversed by better control. As high blood sugars impede the normal process of the white blood cells for attacking bacteria and protecting the body from infection, once the blood sugar returns to normal the will of the white blood cells to fight returns and resistance to infection is restored. This is why controlled diabetics heal well after surgery or injury and are not unduly prone to infections.

High blood sugar (hyperglycemia)

I said before that many diabetics have high blood sugar when their doctor tells them for the first time that they are diabetic. Once you are already on a course of diabetic treatment you can also develop high blood sugar (known as hyperglycemia) through overeating, infections, severe emotional upsets, or sometimes by forgetting to take antidiabetes pills or insulin. Hyperglycemia is caused by the pancreas not making enough insulin to meet your body's requirements. In cases of either hyperglycemia, or low blood sugar known as hypoglycemia, a person will feel ill. A major difference between the symptoms of the two conditions is that hyperglycemia usually takes a few days, sometimes hours, to develop, whereas hypoglycemia can occur within minutes.

Low blood sugar (hypoglycemia)

Hypoglycemia occurs when insulin or antidiabetes pills don't match your food intake. This could occur either if food is not eaten at the regular time after your insulin injection or if unexpected exercise lowers your blood sugar when no other source of food energy is available to the body. During its early stages, mild hypoglycemia is fairly common after meals, and when the blood sugars drop to an abnormally low level the diabetic patient feels unwell. Diabetics not on insulin often produce insulin sluggishly. So after a meal, for example, the pancreas tries to produce enough insulin to meet the increased blood sugar. But the peak is reached too late so by the time the insulin arrives into the blood, the sugar level has already fallen. This late insulin peak causes the blood sugar to drop to an abnormally low level, giving early symptoms of hypoglycemia.

Hypoglycemia can develop suddenly and cause hunger, weakness, sweating, nervousness, numbness and tingling, or pounding of the heart – symptoms due to adrenalin release from the adrenal gland. Hypoglycemia can also cause drowsiness, confusion, loss of memory, headaches or slurred speech, because the brain is not getting enough glucose to function properly. Most diabetics will recognize at least one or two of these symptoms. These hypoglycemic symptoms are usually temporary and disappear without treatment.

Comas (ketoacidosis)

In my hospital about one in four cases of children who develop diabetes is

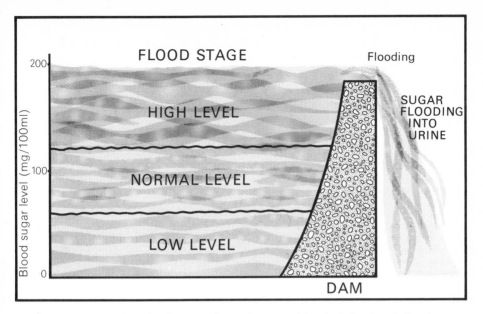

When the water in the lake rises up above the normal level of the dam it floods over. Similarly in the diabetic, when the blood sugar rises above about 180 mg per 100 ml the kidneys are unable to hold the sugar back and it floods over into the urine.

brought in with coma when their diabetes develops. Last year about 20 children were brought in. As well as increasing blood sugars, the lack of insulin in these individuals prevents the complete breakdown of fats in their bodies. Usually fat is either completely burned as energy or stored as layers of fat. In the diabetic, however, fat can't be fully used and fragments, known as ketones or acetone, seep into the blood. As the diabetic is unable to store fats without insulin, ketones continue to accumulate in the blood.

Ketones and acetone are weak acids. As they build up in the blood, a condition called ketoacidosis develops. This is also sometimes known as ketosis by doctors. The earliest signs of ketoacidosis are nausea and a faster rate of breathing. This can later be followed by increased thirst, excessive urination, vomiting or abdominal pain, listlessness and eventually sleepiness, which are all symptoms of acidosis. If ketoacidosis is not recognized early on, it may be followed by coma and loss of consciousness. If the build up of ketones in the blood continues for a few days, or even a few hours, the results are life-threatening.

If any juvenile-type diabetic checks his or her urine carefully every day, has regular meals as suggested by their doctor or dietitian, and has their insulin injections as directed, I can say with confidence that these problems should not occur. If you are not feeling well and your urine tests

19

Comes on rapidly	HIGH BLOOD SUGAR (HYPERGLYCEMIA)
WARNING SIGNS • Anxiety • Faintness • Headache • Trembling • Hunger • Nausea • Heart pounding • Excessive sweating • Rapid pulse • Tiredness • Not able to waken • Irritability **WHAT TO DO** • Take fruit juice, sugar or food containing sugar • Give glucagon if unconscious • Call doctor if severe or frequent • Do not give fluids if patient is unconscious **CAUSES** • Too much insulin • Unusual amount of exercise • Delayed meal • Too little food	**WARNING SIGNS** • Breathing labored and heavy • Drowsiness • Fatigue • Lack of energy • Thirstiness • Urination increase • Large amounts of sugar or ketones in urine **WHAT TO DO** • Call doctor • Take insulin, if directed by doctor • Drink fluids • Continue urine tests **CAUSES** • Too little insulin • Too much food • Infection or fever • Emotional stress
(HYPOGLYCEMIA INSULIN REACTION) LOW BLOOD SUGAR	Comes on slowly

show large amounts of sugar, the urine should also be checked for ketones: this can be done using Acetest® tablets or Ketostix® dipsticks. If the level is high, contact your doctor immediately. If there is ketosis he may advise additional insulin to help get rid of the ketones in your blood. Whenever you feel unwell, such as if you have flu, it is important to remember to keep up your diet program and the insulin injections.

Comas in adult-type diabetics (hyperglycemic comas)

Sometimes also hyperglycemia may be severe enough to cause a coma. Adult-type diabetics rarely have ketoacidosis: due to prolonged build-up of blood sugar they occasionally can develop hyperglycemic coma. At my hospital we treat about 20 patients each year with this condition. Since there are no ketones in the urine to alert you to this problem, you should look for other clues. When your urine shows large amounts of sugar at every test for 48 hours or longer, you could be getting to a danger point. This condition can develop if your diabetes is controlled just by diet, by taking antidiabetes pills or insulin. The persistent presence of sugar in your urine is unhealthy and keeps you on the verge of developing hyperglycemic coma. As there are no ketones in the blood this is also sometimes known as non-ketotic coma.

In non-diabetics, as mentioned before, the blood sugar is always below 150 mg per 100 ml (8 mmol per liter). With this type of coma the blood sugar usually exceeds 800 mg (44 mmol per liter) and may in extreme cases go as high as 4500 mg (200 mmol per liter) – 30 times higher than normal! Such very high blood sugars are only found with badly neglected health, and this condition can develop before the person has realized that he or she has diabetes. Before their blood sugar becomes so extremely high, most people will already have been ill for weeks or even months.

If you already have diabetes, two problems may set off this condition – an illness such as the flu (either respiratory or stomach flu), or starting on a new medication. Medicines which may worsen your diabetes are steroid hormones (such as prednisone), pills to increase urine flow (diuretics), pills for high blood pressure and some other drugs. As well as high sugars in the urine, you should be alert in case you get very thirsty, start to urinate far more than usual, especially during the night, or if you get unusually tired. Careful measurement of your urine sugar tests will help you to avoid this problem.

I have included the following example as I think it provides an interesting illustration of the unlikely way some diabetics can first learn of their condition. This is how Walter first developed diabetes at fifty-six years old.

His blood sugar level had become incredibly high before he started to notice anything was wrong. He started to drink more and more fluids. He was always thirsty. As he worked as a roofer this became very awkward for him. Walter had to come down off the roof almost every 30 minutes and drink one or two coca colas. He took twelve cokes to work and kept them in a cooler in his truck. He also lost over 30 lb (13.5 kg) and had to urinate three or four times during the night. Although he had much less energy than usual he still managed to carry on working for over three months in spite of these problems.

One very hot day, however, it became just too much for him. He finished his last coke at lunch. He worked for two hours after lunch fixing a roof. Then he moved over unsteadily to the ladder, came down it slowly and collapsed under a tree. His assistant rushed over to him and Walter had passed out. An emergency squad brought him to our hospital. His blood sugar was over 2000 mg per 100 ml (110 mmol per liter) and he was very dehydrated. A combination of cola drinks and excessive sweating had shot his blood sugar up and dried him out. Except for his diabetes Walter was strong as an ox.

We treated him with insulin and gave him fluids into the veins to rehydrate him. Within six hours he was again eating and drinking normally. We brought his blood sugar back down to normal within four days with daily insulin injections. He recovered very well and returned to work ten days later. For several months Walter took his insulin daily. We slowly reduced the dose and four months after he first developed diabetes he came off insulin therapy.

He now follows our high fiber diet very carefully and his diabetes is well controlled without insulin or pills. An awareness of the common warning signs of diabetes might have alerted Walter to the possibility that he had the disease and brought him in to see us earlier.

2 KEEPING YOUR BLOOD SUGAR ON TARGET

How to control your diabetes

Consistency, regularity and moderation are the features of well-managed diabetes. You should control your diabetes, instead of letting it control you. To do this you and your doctor must work out a plan together to include a diet, an insulin program (if required) and an exercise plan. Consistency in terms of insulin injections or taking antidiabetes pills, regularity of mealtimes so that your body can adjust to a routine, and moderation in work, stress and food are necessary. In short, as you develop better discipline, your diabetes will be better controlled. You can be more flexible, but only if you have your diabetes under good control. Disregarding your diabetes may give you some temporary freedom but the disease will eventually take control over your life again.

Your doctor plays an important role in helping you regulate your diabetes. You and he should work closely with each other as two partners on the same team. You'll have to keep careful daily records of your urine sugar tests, medications including insulin injections, antidiabetes pills taken, and general health. Your blood will also have to be tested at a laboratory from time to time. Your doctor may also want you to check your own blood sugar at home.

Having diabetes is a nuisance – there are no books entitled *The Joy of Diabetes*. Any diabetic can list many drawbacks such as taking injections, testing urine, avoiding having sweets and candies. This handicap, though, can be turned into an advantage. Success has been achieved by many people because of a handicap. In having to initially force themselves to overcome it they have developed a determination that has helped them achieve success.

You can actually become a healthier person because you have diabetes. As you will be forced to take good care of your condition you develop healthy habits such as a well-balanced diet and regular exercise. Diabetes itself is not a major health hazard; and if you control it you can prevent possible serious consequences such as heart disease and stroke.

Towards better health

The following discipline, if stuck to carefully, can lead to a healthier and longer life.

1. Take meticulous care of your diabetes. This includes taking your insulin or pills on time, eating your meals at the scheduled times, regularly checking your urine for glucose, and keeping the careful records recommended by your doctor.
2. Eat a wholesome diet that helps you control the disease and lowers your blood fats.
3. Keep up a healthy exercise program.
4. Control your own schedule – do not let it control you. You must get enough sleep. Do not work excessively long hours.
5. Diabetics are at risk for coronary heart disease. You should use moderation in the amount of alcohol you drink, the food you eat, exercise you take and also avoid working too hard, mental stress and tiring yourself out. As smoking is a major risk factor causing heart attack and stroke, it is advisable to cut out smoking altogether.

NAME _____   DIET _____

GLUCOSE TESTS							
Date	Weight	Before breakfast	Before noon meal	Before evening meal	At bedtime	Insulin dose a.m./p.m.	Comments (Insulin reactions?)

Keep a daily record on a sheet like the one above of your glucose tests and insulin doses, as well as other useful information, to show your doctor on your next check-up.

6. Uncontrolled high blood pressure can also lead to heart attack or stroke. Regular check-ups should also lead to earlier detection and treatment of high blood pressure.

All the above measures should reduce the likelihood of developing a heart attack or a stroke. Although only the first one relates specifically to your diabetes, the remaining points are directed at maintaining good general health.

Control of diabetes is a balancing act

As a diabetic you must achieve a good balance between low and high blood sugars as either of these can cause comas. While food raises the blood sugar, insulin and exercise lower it. Your aim is to achieve a balance between these so that your blood sugar stays in a satisfactory range at all times. This is where a schedule or discipline comes into play. It is also the point where you must make daily decisions without direct advice from your doctor.

Your schedule should involve meals and snacks taken at regular times, day in and day out. Although it can be monotonous this discipline is especially important for control of your diabetes if you take insulin or pills. I feel strongly that sticking to a diet program and eating regularly every day is your primary building block for better diabetic control. Breakfast should be taken at the same time each day. Every day your breakfast should have the same number of food exchanges (this is a process of exchanging one kind of food for another of the same type, for instance, milk, breakfast cereals, fruit, bread – see chapter nine for a full explanation).

This also applies to both your midday and evening meals. Whether you are on one, two or three snacks a day, you should try to take them at the same time each day. If your amount of exercise varies, you may vary the amount of food at certain snacks under the guidance of your doctor or dietitian.

Control over your diabetes is like a stool supported by three legs – diet, exercise, and insulin or pills (if required). If one leg breaks you lose control of your diabetes. So diet, for example, is just as important as your insulin injections.

Checking your blood sugar

Urine tests
Most of my patients test their own urine for sugar three or four times every day, the results helping them to adjust their own treatment.

Test paper tapes (Tes-Tape®) remain yellow if there is no sugar in the urine; after 60 seconds these strips turn green or blue if sugar is present. There is a color chart on the box. Light green represents $\frac{1}{10}$ per cent glucose, dark green is $\frac{1}{4}$ per cent, dark green to blue is $\frac{1}{2}$ per cent, and dark blue is 2 per cent or more sugar. Tes-Tapes® are not available in Britain and are not commonly used in Australia.

To use Clinitest® tablets you need to collect your urine in a clean container. Place five drops of urine and ten drops of water in a test tube, and drop one tablet into the tube. Watch the tube while the boiling takes place. Wait 15 seconds after the boiling has stopped and gently shake the tube to completely mix the contents. Ignore any sediment at the bottom of the tube and compare the color of the liquid with the color chart. If there is no sugar, the solution is blue. A green color represents $\frac{1}{4}$ per cent glucose, a cloudy green is $\frac{1}{2}$ per cent, an olive green is $\frac{3}{4}$ per cent, a yellow to light brown is 1 per cent and an orange is 2 per cent. Watching the tube during the boiling period and afterwards shows you the 'pass through' color changes which occur when the urine has more than 2 per cent sugar. The color rapidly passes through bright orange to a dark brown or greenish-brown color. If this occurs frequently you should use the two-drop Clinitest® method. In Britain Clinitest® is the long-standing method of urine testing.

The two-drop Clinitest® method can be used to check the sugar in single urine samples, or to measure glucose loss in the urine over a 12 or 24-hour period. This test extends the range 2 per cent to 5 per cent. You will need to get a special chart for the two-drop test. If no glucose is present in the urine, the liquid will be blue. A green color represents $\frac{1}{4}$ per cent glucose, cloudy green is $\frac{1}{2}$ per cent, olive green is 1 per cent, yellowish brown is 2 per cent, light brown is 3 per cent and orange is 5 per cent or more. With the two-drop method you can find out how much sugar you spill in a day, by collecting all your urine over a 24-hour period. Many diabetics find collection of their urine over a 24-hour period rather inconvenient and they can sometimes forget to take a urine sample. Some clinics use the two-drop method for greater accuracy when testing children's urine.

Sometimes I use the following short-cut for the Clinitest® method. I get my patients to collect all their urine from 7 pm to 7 am. After the evening meal you empty your bladder just before 7 pm and throw this urine away. Save all urine passed after 7 pm and empty your bladder again at 7 am; save this specimen. Pour all urine into a measuring container to get the number of milliliters. Test the urine with the two-drop Clinitest®. If the test reads 1 per cent and your urine volume is 1000 ml you have spilled 10 g of sugar – 1 per cent 1000 ml = 10 ml or 10 g. If you spill less than 5 g between 7 pm and 7 am you are doing well.

Many diabetics prefer using dipsticks (Diastix®). The advantages are that you don't need to collect your urine and also you don't need to boil anything. As strip tests are more convenient than tablets they are rapidly increasing in popularity in Britain and are already commonly used in North America and Australia.

When there is no sugar in the urine Diastix® remain blue for 30 seconds. A green or brown color indicates the presence of sugar. Light green represents $\frac{1}{10}$ per cent glucose, dark green is $\frac{1}{4}$ per cent, olive green is $\frac{1}{2}$ per cent, light brown is 1 per cent and dark brown is 2 per cent (2 per cent glucose is 2 g of glucose per 100 ml – 111 mmol per liter). When making this test, it is very important to remember to wait for a full 30 seconds before checking the color of the Diastix®.

Direct blood sugar tests

Home tests   Until recently my patients and I used urine sugar records and intermittent blood sugar measurements taken in the laboratory (see below) to assess their diabetic control. With the practical techniques now available for measuring blood sugars at home, we can tell how high the blood sugar actually is at certain times during the day. More importantly, we can also tell how low it drops and how much fast-acting sugar must be eaten to bring it back to normal. This is much more accurate than urine tests. Insulin doses can be adjusted much more intelligently and the whole treatment including diet and exercise programs can be more confidently planned using this information.

To obtain your own blood sugar reading only a single drop of your blood is needed. I recommend the following technique: hold your hand down at your side for several minutes or under warm running water so blood flows to the finger; wipe the fingertip with alcohol-based cleansing solution and allow it to dry completely; use a Monolet® with a plastic guard to prevent you from going too deep. Many patients who don't like having to prick themselves prefer to use the Autolet® Lancet, which automatically pricks your fingertip after you push the release.

With a minimal amount of 'milking' a drop of blood will form at the puncture site. The first drop can be directly transferred to the chemical strip for measuring the blood sugar.

The Chemstrip bG® is a chemical strip which can be used for a visual reading without a special machine. This is known as the BM-Test Glycemie 20-800 in Britain and Australia. Using this, the approximate

27

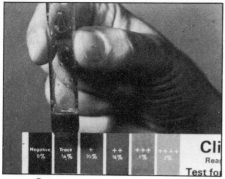

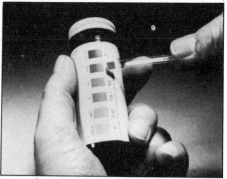

Clintest® Wait 15 seconds after boiling the urine in a clean container. Shake the contents then check the color.

Diastix® When there is no glucose in the urine Diastix® remain blue for 30 seconds.

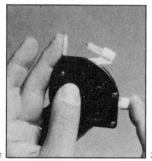

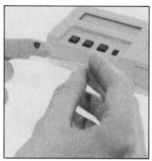

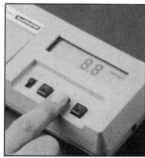

Glucometer® 1. The finger can be pricked using an Autolet®. 2. A drop of blood is put on a Dextrostix® for exactly 60 seconds. The strip is then washed and blotted dry, and put into the monitor to be read. 3. The blood sugar reading shown on the digital panel is measured here in mmol per liter. It is equivalent to 158 mg per 100 ml.

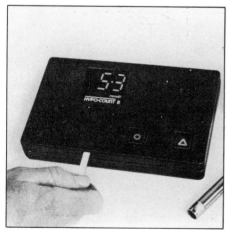

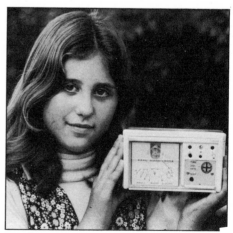

Hypo-Count B® This portable, blood glucose monitor is compatible with BM-Test Glycemie strips.

GEM® This particular machine was developed in Australia (where it is called the RAHC glucose tester) by Stan Clark to help his diabetic daughter (above).

blood sugar can be read from a chart on the pack.

To use Dextrostix® chemical strips you will need an electrically operated blood glucose monitor. Use of these blood glucose monitors has been growing in popularity. The Dextrometer® is now well established in North America but other similar models are on the market which can either be plugged in to the main electricity or use a rechargeable battery pack. To use either a Dextrometer® or the Glucometer® you need to use calibration strips or fluid to standardize your machine (see opposite). The trend has been for use of smaller, portable home monitors such as the Glucometer® which is now available in most countries. Its batteries last for 1000 tests, usually about one year's use. Other models available in Britain include the Glucochek® monitor (which is also compatible with Dextrostix®), the Hypo-Count® and the GEM® (known in Australia as the RAHC tester).

When you buy a new bottle of Dextrostix®, you will need to restandardize your machine using a fresh Dextrostix®, and the glucose test solution. As long as you leave your machine plugged in you don't need to use another Dextrostix®. Each day you should recheck your machine by using the calibration strips, and if the strip gives you a reading of within 10 per cent of the calibrated values (80 to 100 mg per 100 ml for the 90 mg per 100 ml calibration strip) your machine is set for use.

Two other strips are also now available from the manufacturers of Chemstrip bG® (BM-Test Glycemie 20-800) for use in conjunction with some monitors. The Reflotest Hypoglycemie® measures a low level of blood sugar and the Reflotest Glucose®, normal to upper levels.

Laboratory tests   The concentration of sugar in the blood can also be measured directly in a laboratory. Usually the sugar is measured in plasma, which is the part of the blood that does not contain red and white blood cells. This is why the test is known as a plasma glucose test. Red blood cells carry oxygen to body tissues using a vital protein called hemoglobin. Whenever the blood sugar becomes too high, many proteins throughout the body, including hemoglobin, are sugar-coated. In the laboratory, the amount of sugar attached to hemoglobin is measured; this test is called the glycohemoglobin or sugar-hemoglobin test. I use it to estimate how many times and for how long during the previous six-week period the blood sugar has been excessively high.

What is good control?

You have good control when the urine sugar tests taken four times per day have no sugar at least 95 per cent of the time, the fasting and three-hours-after-meal plasma sugar values are less than 150 mg per 100 ml (8 mmol per liter), and the glycohemoglobin value is less than 10 per cent in my laboratory. This degree of control can rarely be achieved for juvenile-type diabetics without using insulin infusion pumps (see chapter ten). Most diabetics, however, can achieve good control with either diet alone, or diet with either pills or insulin.

Your own diet

I said before that diet, insulin and exercise are the three 'legs' supporting the diabetes 'stool'. Before you developed diabetes, your pancreas made enough insulin to keep your blood sugar normal at all times. If you ate six or eight times a day, your own insulin met the challenge. Every time you ate, your pancreas sent out the correct amount of insulin to match your body's needs. Even if you ate an entire apple pie, your pancreas could still match the insulin to stabilize the blood sugar. Now, as a diabetic, you may depend on one or two injections of insulin every day, so the tables are turned. You must now eat to match your insulin injections instead of having your own insulin match your food intake.

Whatever type of diabetes you have, diet is your most important weapon against the disease. So don't think that if you don't take insulin then this part of the book doesn't really apply to you. It applies if you take pills, if you are just on a special diet or have borderline diabetes. In any kind of diabetes the beta-cells do not produce enough insulin; your pancreas does not make enough to keep your blood sugar at a normal level. If, for instance, you eat two big pieces of chocolate cake with icing and drink a large Coca Cola®, your pancreas gives up – there is no way that it can release enough insulin to restrain the rise of your blood sugar. So whether you take insulin or not, you have to eat properly so that your insulin can keep your blood sugar within a healthy range.

What your diet should do for you

If you have diabetes, you should expect your own diet to do two things for you. First, it should help you keep your blood sugar and blood fats within a healthy range, so reducing your chances of developing complications of diabetes such as hardening of the arteries and heart attack. Second, your diet should provide you with all the necessary nutrients. If you are overweight, your diet should help you to lose weight, keeping you in the healthiest condition possible. You should ask yourself the question 'What is my diet doing for me?' If the answer is that you don't know, perhaps you should reconsider your diet plan.

Setting goals for your own diet

If your diet is going to help you, it needs to be carefully planned. You must work closely with both your doctor and dietitian. A diet sheet, even a sample diet included in this book, won't work. Every diabetic needs a diet tailormade for his or her special needs. This book can give you guidelines for developing your own diet, but unless you have had special training, you will need the help of your doctor or dietitian.

If you take insulin, your diet must meet several special needs. First, it should work with the insulin to keep your blood sugar within a healthy range after meals. Second, it should prevent you from having insulin reactions. Third, it should provide the energy you need for both work and exercise. In addition to your three main meals, you need between one and three snacks a day.

I recommend snacks for my patients as follows: if they take, for example, a single dose of NPH (Isophane) or Lente insulin (see the next chapter), they will need to eat a snack at bedtime (some also need a midafternoon snack to prevent low blood sugars). If they take a combination of regular (soluble) and NPH (Isophane) in the morning, they need to have a midmorning snack. I recommend a minimum of three snacks a day for children, patients taking two insulin injections a day, and for very active people. Meals and snacks act as a balance for insulin injections and exercise. Most of my patients have three meals and a bedtime snack every day.

If you take antidiabetes pills (see next chapter), diet and exercise will help you avoid 'the needle'. Overeating puts a strain on the pancreas and may lead to exhaustion. Moderation in eating is the best way to keep your pancreas working.

If you are overweight, you have been overeating. Following your diet will help you lose 1 to 2 lb ($\frac{1}{2}$ to 1 kg) in weight each week. Exercise also helps you lose weight. When you overeat your blood sugar becomes too high and sugar spills into the urine. One way to correct this problem is to take more insulin, but this is the wrong way. The right way is to stop overeating. If you are on a large dose of insulin (over 40 units per day), it will be difficult for you to decrease your food intake without decreasing your insulin dose; you may have to overeat to avoid low blood sugars.

So you and your doctor, together with the help of his team, need to develop a plan for decreasing both your insulin dose and your food intake at the same time. With weight loss, most of my more overweight patients with less severe diabetes can gradually decrease their insulin dose, and

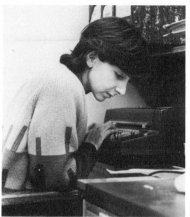

Typing uses 100 calories.

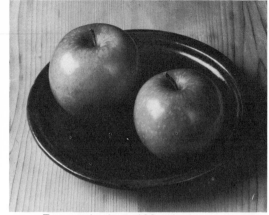

Two apples have 100 calories.

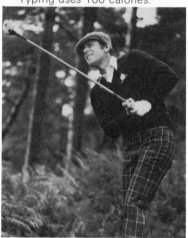

Playing golf uses 150 calories.

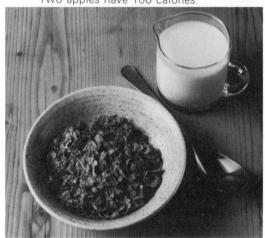

Cereal and skim milk has 150 calories.

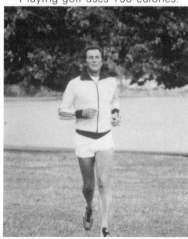

Running uses 300 calories.

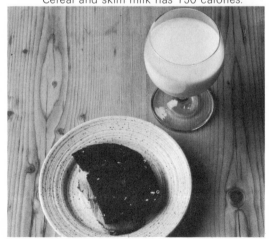

A roast-beef sandwich has 300 calories.

Activity, calories and food equivalents

Activity (for 30 minutes)	Calories	Food Equivalent (each item)

LIGHT

Bicycling (5 mph)	100*	Wholewheat bread (2 slices)
Bowling		Wholewheat roll (1 small slice) with
House painting		margarine
Ironing or sewing		Banana (large)
Table tennis		Apples (2 medium)
Typing		Grape juice (1 cup)
Volley ball		Milk, 1% (1 cup)
Walking slowly (2½ mph)		

MODERATE

Dancing	150*	Turkey sandwich: turkey (1 oz); bread (2
Gardening		slices)
Golf		Cereal (1 serving) and skim milk (1 cup)
Lawn mowing		Beans, brown (½ cup, 3 oz) and corn bread
Scrubbing floors		(1 square)
Tennis		Grape juice (1 cup)
Walking rapidly (3½ mph)		

HEAVY

Basketball	300*	Roast beef (2 oz) on rye or wholewheat
Cycling (13 mph)		bread (2 slices) with skim milk (1 cup)
Digging ditch		Spaghetti (1 cup, 2 oz) with meat sauce
Football		and bread (1 slice)
Running		Bean soup (large bowl) with rye crackers
Shovelling snow		or crispbread (3)
Squash or handball		
Swimming		

*In some countries the new system of kilojoules (kJ) is used. The calories given will be 420 kJ, 630 kJ and 1260 kJ. Australian readers should substitute 300 ml skim milk or 150 ml milk for 1 cup 1% milk and 1 metric cup (250 ml) grape juice.

LEFT: The number of calories used by a 150 lb (70 kg) person doing the activity shown for 30 minutes. The equivalent number of food calories is given above.

some can stop their insulin injections completely. I must emphasize that no diabetic should ever consider making any major change in their current treatment program without first consulting their doctor. Under no circumstances should any diabetic on insulin try to give it up except with the full knowledge and supervision of his or her doctor.

What exercise can do for you

Exercise is the second leg supporting you in control over your diabetes. It lowers your blood sugar and reduces your need for insulin or pills. Somehow, exercise makes insulin work better on your muscle and fat cells. Exercise lowers your blood fats and probably decreases your chance of having a heart attack. In general, your circulation improves and your blood vessels are healthier if you exercise regularly. Some people find that exercise also relieves tension and leads to better health and even to a feeling of euphoria.

If you are in good physical shape, active in sports and under thirty years old, you can develop your own exercise program. You should ask your doctor for his or her advice about your insulin dose and eating extra food before exercising. Some of my patients take slightly less regular (soluble) insulin (see next chapter) before a period of strenuous exercise such as before a sports event or even before running. Others eat extra carbohydrate before, during and after the exercise. The table on page 33 gives a guide to the amount of food needed to sustain certain common exercises. In general if your urine tests show no sugar or only small amounts, exercise will lower your blood sugar. If, on the other hand you have moderate or large amounts of sugar or ketones in your urine, exercise alone will not lower your blood sugar. Adequate amounts of insulin will also be required as well as the exercise. So don't be put off if you can't improve a 2 per cent test for urine glucose with a long spell of running.

Several of my patients have told me that they don't get low blood sugar while jogging; but they do seem to develop low blood sugar while resting after a run. Recent research suggests that the blood sugar seems to be autoregulated during exercise. This means that the body tends to protect you from a low blood sugar during exercise. After you have finished your exercise session, you may then be subject to the effects of a low blood sugar. Nevertheless, you must take precautions before and during exercise, and always have some fast-acting sugar with you. After the age of thirty, most of us become less physically active than we were during the earlier years of our life, and because of changes in eating habits and exercise patterns most of us gain weight.

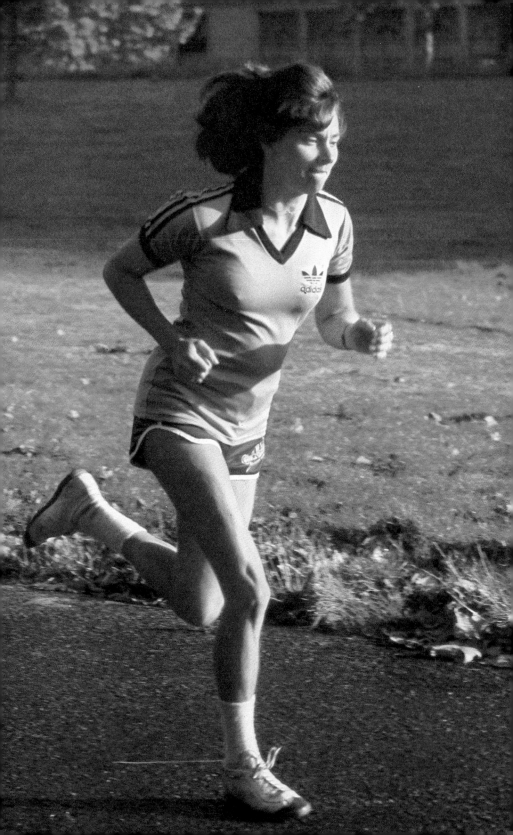

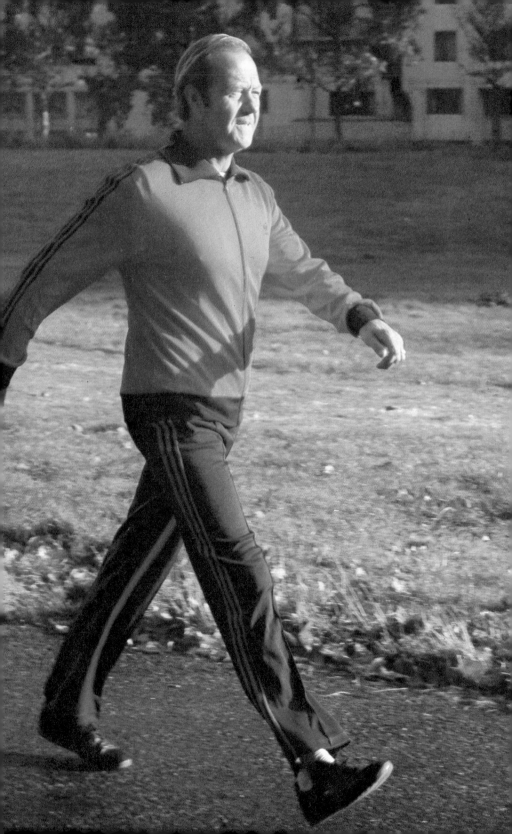

Taking up physical exercise is both a good way to restore health and to lose weight. I recommend walking as the exercise of choice for diabetic patients over thirty. If you want to jog, first check with your doctor. He may want to give you a checkup by taking an electrocardiogram test during and after your exercise; this is to measure the capacity of your heart to support moderate amounts of exercise. But whether you walk, jog, run or swim you should begin slowly and use common sense. If you have been inactive for a long time, you should begin by walking a comfortable distance twice a day. It may take you perhaps 25 to 30 minutes to walk 1 mile ($1\frac{1}{2}$ km). Don't get discouraged and don't rush your programme. I recommend maintaining the same schedule for the first six days, with one day of rest each week.

When you begin the second week, try to walk about 20 per cent further each day than you did the first week. Remember that distance is more important than time. Each week you should try to walk about 20 per cent further each day than you did the last week. As you gain strength you may be able to cut down on the time required. The aim is to walk briskly for about 30 minutes twice daily. You will thus be walking between 3 and 4 miles (5 and $6\frac{1}{2}$ km) daily, 6 days a week.

If you develop chest pain (angina), pain in your arms or shoulders, have moderate difficulty in breathing, or leg pain (claudication) you should consult your doctor about your exercise program. I have found a sensible walking program to be very safe for my patients, as it does not lead to the physical trauma commonly associated with jogging or running. Walking, however, requires more time to achieve an optimal health benefit. But don't you think your health is worth the investment? If you can walk briskly approximately 15 miles (24 km) a week during your designated walking times, this is probably adequate to develop and sustain a beneficial effect on your heart function. This 15 miles, however, does *not* include the distance you cover while meandering to work or ambling through a shopping center.

Among my patients, I have found that an active exercise program coupled with a high-carbohydrate, high-fiber, low-fat diet leads to improved circulation to the heart and the legs. In hospitalized patients chest pain frequently improves or disappears on our diet and exercise program. Leg pain diminishes and some patients can walk five to ten times further without pain after being on this program for three to six weeks. Research is beginning to show improvement or reversal of hardening of the arteries with diet and exercise programs.

3 USING INSULIN AND ANTIDIABETES PILLS PROPERLY

The third 'leg' in a good diabetic program is your course of insulin injections, if you need them. Insulin is a miracle drug. Since its discovery in 1921, it has saved countless lives, and today it helps millions of diabetics lead healthy and productive lives.

Before 1921, when a child developed diabetes, the consequences were similar to a fast-growing cancer. The child lost weight rapidly and had very little chance of surviving for even two years. Dr Bragg, one of my professors when I was a medical student, developed diabetes in 1921 at the age of fourteen years old to the considerable alarm and grief of his parents. Fortunately for Dr Bragg, insulin became available within nine months of his developing diabetes and he was able to resume a full and active life. He became one of the leading teachers and physicians in the diabetes field. Sixty years after its discovery insulin still has to be taken as an injection but this is a minor annoyance compared to its tremendous benefits.

The key to good use of insulin is finding the correct dose that corresponds to your blood sugar changes produced by the amount of food you eat and your level of physical activity. In other words, your blood insulin level should be high when your blood sugar is high, and both should be low at the same time. You will need to work closely with your doctor and health care team to perfect an insulin program which meets your own specific needs. In this chapter I will give you some basic information about insulin and then show how my patients and I work together to find the best insulin doses to meet their own individual needs.

The different types of insulin

Diabetes is commonly treated by two general types of insulin – fast-acting or slow-acting. Regular insulin, known as soluble insulin outside North America, is a pure preparation which does not contain any added proteins or zinc to modify or alter its action. When injected subcutaneously (into the fat under the skin) regular (soluble) insulin starts to act in about half an hour, has its peak or maximum effect in two to three hours, and a duration of action of about six hours. Other insulin preparations are modified by the addition of protein or zinc to extend their duration of action.

NPH (known as Isophane outside North America) and Lente insulin are both slow-acting types which begin to act about two to three hours after a subcutaneous injection. They have a peak of between eight and sixteen hours after injection, and a duration of action of about twenty-four hours.

Semilente insulin is similar to regular (soluble) insulin but has a slightly longer duration of action. Ultralente and protamine-zinc (PZI) insulins are very slow-acting, with a duration of action of about 36 hours.

In many countries, monocomponent, highly purified insulins are becoming popular. Their main advantages are: they are less likely to lead to reactions at local injection sites, patients often need to take smaller doses of insulin, and insulin antibodies are less likely to occur (see page 51). The insulins are known by their brand names. Patients should never switch from one type of insulin to another except as instructed by their doctor.

Insulin is usually obtained from the pancreas of cows and pigs. Most insulin preparations are a mixture of beef and pork insulins, although pure beef and pure pork insulins are available. Pure pork insulin is less likely to produce allergic side-effects.

The new insulins contain 100 units of insulin per milliliter. This is called U100 insulin. So if you take 50 units of U100 insulin you are taking $\frac{1}{2}$ ml. U40 and U80 insulins are no longer available in the United States but are still used in Britain and some other countries. For special needs U500 (500 units per ml) and other strengths of insulin can be used.

How do you know when insulin has its strongest effect?

The effects of insulin depend on the type of insulin, your eating habits and physical exercise patterns. You should know yourself when your insulin is having its strongest effects. Try to always take your meals and exercise at regular times every day. If you delay the time when you usually have your meal slightly you can sometimes start to feel unwell. If this happens and your urine test shows no sugar in your urine, this will show that your insulin doses are acting strongly.

Your urine tests for sugar will always provide you with the first clue to when your insulin is acting. There should be no sugar in the urine (0 per cent or negative) when your insulin is having its strongest effect. The timing of your reactions gives you another clue. Most should occur when your insulin is at its peak activity. So, if you take NPH (Isophane) insulin

Effect of insulin on blood sugar

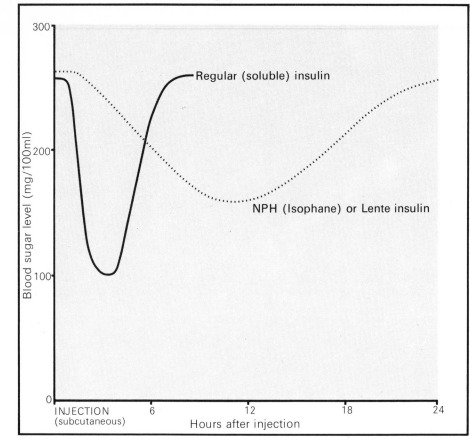

This shows when insulin has its peak activity.

in the morning for example, it is likely to have its strongest effects before your evening meal. Most of your urine tests should be negative (o per cent sugar) and you should feel the effects more frequently at this time. When you realize this, you can take better precautions if your evening meal is delayed or you do unaccustomed exercise at this time.

If your diabetes is not adequately controlled, it may be difficult for you to find out when your insulin is having its strongest effects. If you don't keep to consistent meals and exercise, you may find that your urine isn't free of sugar often enough for you to be able to check the best time of day to take your insulin injections. If you use two different types of insulin, or take two injections a day, you will obviously find it harder to work out when each one is having its strongest effect. But take the trouble to find out when your insulin is acting at its strongest. Once you have learned this you will find it much easier to master your diabetes. Care in taking your urine tests and recording of the results are also really worth the effort.

Insulin reactions (low blood sugar)
If you do take insulin, your dose has been carefully prescribed for you by your doctor to use up the correct amount of sugar after you have eaten your meals. But if you miss a meal for some reason or you use far more energy than usual due to intensive or uncharacteristically high levels of physical exercise, your normal dose of insulin can cause your blood sugar to drop too low. This is also known as an insulin reaction, and if left unchecked can culminate in hypoglycemia or even coma.

A hypoglycemic insulin reaction (often called a 'hypo' by diabetics) can develop, for example, as a result of taking too much insulin or even too many antidiabetes pills, not eating enough food through missing a meal, leaving too much time between taking insulin and eating, or doing an unusual amount of exercise. When the blood sugar is low there will be no sugar in the urine.

If you get an insulin reaction the simplest way to overcome it is by eating some fast-acting sugar. You'll feel better almost immediately. Because of this risk diabetics should always keep an emergency supply of sugar handy – perhaps in the car glove compartment, or in a handbag. Other solid carbohydrate foods such as bread do not act quickly enough. If the insulin reaction has led to loss of consciousness, it could take 15 minutes or longer to recover; the longer the condition is left untreated, the more potentially damaging it can be, possibly needing a doctor to give an emergency glucose injection. So if you ever suspect you may have any of the early symptoms described above, you just take some sugar or a sweetened drink however mild the symptoms may seem. The more you know about your diabetes, the better you can regulate your own blood sugar.

Adjusting your own dose of insulin
Many doctors give their patients instructions for adjusting their own insulin doses. Your doctor can give you advice based on your own special insulin needs.

I instruct my patients using the following general guidelines. Take, for example, a patient on two injections a day. He takes NPH (Isophane) and regular (soluble) insulin before breakfast and before the evening meal. If he has 1 or 2 per cent sugar in his urine before lunch on several consecutive days he *increases* his morning regular (soluble) insulin dose by two units a day. On the other hand, if he has an insulin reaction before lunch that he can't relate either to an unusual amount of exercise or eating less food than usual, he *reduces* his morning regular (soluble) insulin by two units per day. This is why I ask patients to watch carefully for sugar in their urine or insulin reactions four times a day – before breakfast, before the midday meal, before the evening meal and at bedtime. Now that more of my patients are measuring their own blood sugar at home, we adjust insulin doses as outlined below on the basis of the blood sugar.

I advise my patients that if they get unexplained insulin reactions they should first ask themselves whether this could have been caused by an unusual amount of exercise or by eating less food than usual. Also whether they have recorded 1 or 2 per cent sugar in their urine. If none of these has been responsible, I tell them to adjust their insulin doses, usually by two units. They only change their dose every three days, and they change only one dose at a time, such as the morning NPH (Isophane).

If they have any questions they call me. With these guidelines many of my patients can fine-tune their diabetes between visits. When they have gained experience in adjusting their insulin dose, they can change it to anticipate changes in activity. (For example, if an office worker is going to be much more active on Saturday, he will take less regular (soluble) or NPH (Isophane) insulin on Saturday morning.)

Taking more than one insulin injection a day
Some juvenile-type diabetics whose pancreas makes no insulin at all must take two injections a day to control their diabetes. I try to design an insulin program for each of my patients that keeps the blood sugar within a healthy range for them. This can sometimes be achieved with one dose a day, and sometimes with a mixture of two insulins. Many patients need two injections a day. I find that most of my lean juvenile-type patients need two injections a day, usually a mixture of NPH (Isophane) and regular (soluble) insulin in the morning, and NPH (Isophane) or NPH (Isophane) plus regular (soluble) insulin in the evening.

These insulins usually have their strongest actions as follows:

1. The morning regular (soluble) insulin covers breakfast and keeps the blood sugar and urine sugar within a desirable range before the midday meal.
2. The morning NPH (Isophane) covers the midday meal and keeps the blood sugar and urine sugar within a good range before the evening meal.
3. The evening regular (soluble) is taken before the evening meal and covers the evening meal and keeps the blood and urine sugars within

a good range at bedtime.

4. The evening NPH (Isophane) covers the bedtime snack and maintains a blood insulin level throughout the night.

The following case history shows when a two-injection program is necessary.

Lloyd, a fifty-three year-old juvenile-type diabetic had three different part-time jobs and didn't have time to take two injections of insulin. Lloyd found he was always tired, his urine and blood sugar tests always showed readings that were too high and he was 20 lb (9 kg) underweight. We arranged for him to come into the hospital during a slack period at his work to adjust his insulin program. We started him on a second injection and his diabetes was much better controlled. Within ten days he returned to all three of his jobs. He felt much better having two injections a day, he started gaining weight and tests have shown much better urine and blood sugar levels.

Practical hints for insulin users

Where to inject your insulin

Insulin should be injected into many different parts of the body, such as the thighs or the upper part of the legs, the buttocks, abdomen, and upper arms. You shouldn't inject your insulin into the same areas every day because this will lead to hard lumpy areas or scarring under the skin, and the insulin will not be absorbed well from these damaged places. To avoid these problems you should rotate your injection sites.

For example, during the first week you can give your insulin at a different place on the right thigh; each injection should be at least an inch (25 mm) from the previous injection. During the second week you can use the left thigh, during the third week the right side of the abdomen and so on. By using a rotation plan you will not have to use the same small injection area more than a few times each year, and this will provide you with more consistent day-to-day action from your insulin.

Storing the insulin

Keep the insulin bottle that you are currently using at room temperature. As a general rule, your insulin is comfortable at whatever temperature you are – neither you nor your insulin can tolerate the glove compartment of your car or staying in a stuffy, parked car in hot summer weather. Extra bottles should be kept in the refrigerator until the day before use. Do not use insulin beyond the expiry action date printed on the box.

Drawing insulin

British readers Please turn to page 46

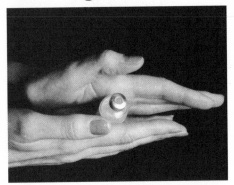

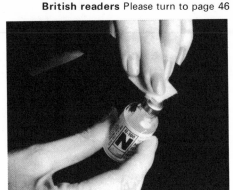

1. After first thoroughly washing your hands, mix insulin completely by gently rolling bottle between your hands. Never shake the insulin.

2. Clean the top of the insulin bottle with an alcohol swab.

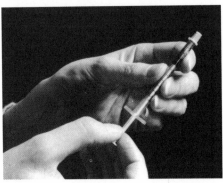

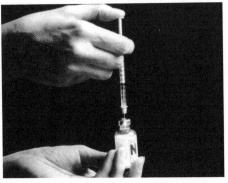

3. Draw same amount of air into syringe as the insulin dose you require.

4. With the bottle upright, insert needle into rubber stopper and push plunger down.

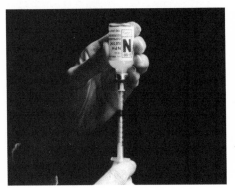

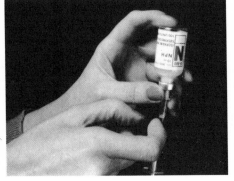

5. Turn the bottle and syringe upside down. Slowly draw up slightly more insulin than your dose.

6. If there are any air bubbles in the syringe, flick or tap at the bubble. When it goes to the top of the syringe push the plunger until the bubble goes into the bottle. Draw your exact dose again.

Injecting insulin

British readers Please turn to page 47

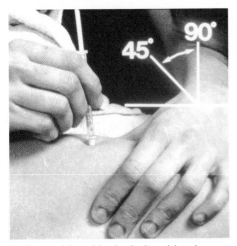

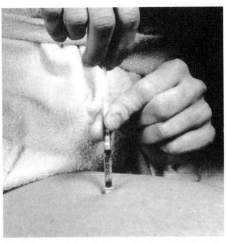

1. Clean skin with alcohol and let dry. Grasp same area between your thumb and fingers, raising skin and fat away from muscle. Hold syringe as shown and inject needle quickly into skin at an angle of 45 to 90°.

2. Release skin. Pull back plunger about 2 or 3 units. Make sure there is no blood in syringe. If there is blood, *don't inject* as it means the needle is in a blood vessel. Throw syringe away and start again.

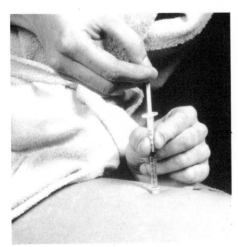

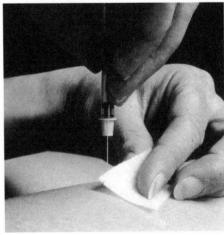

3. Push plunger down quickly and steadily in 3 to 5 seconds.

4. Quickly pull needle from the skin and gently hold an alcohol swab on the injection site to close opening left by needle. Don't massage area.

The British method of drawing insulin

The following is the generally accepted method of drawing and injecting insulin in Britain. The majority of diabetics in Britain use a glass syringe.

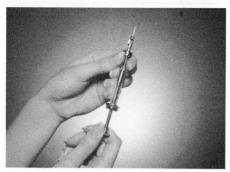

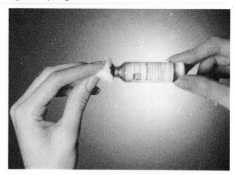

1. Wash hands thoroughly and dry on clean towel. Remove syringe, with needle attached, from its case. Move plunger up and down several times to remove any industrial methylated spirit.

2. Clean cap of insulin bottle with industrial methylated spirit.

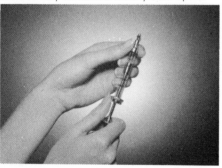

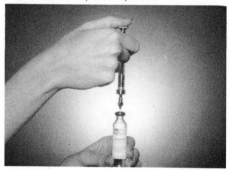

3. Draw same amount of air into syringe as the insulin dose you require.

4. With bottle upright, insert needle through rubber cap, pushing air into the space above the liquid. If you use cloudy, longer-acting insulin, shake bottle gently by up-ending several times before pushing air into the bottle.

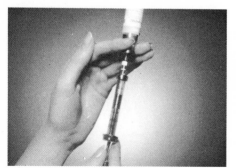

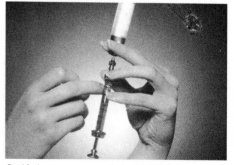

5. Turn bottle and syringe upside down. Make sure that the tip of the needle is well below the surface of the liquid. Slowly draw up your required dose.

6. If there are any air bubbles in syringe, flick or tap at the bubble with your finger. When bubble goes to the top of the syringe, push plunger until you see bubbles go into the bottle. Draw more insulin slowly.

The British method of injecting insulin

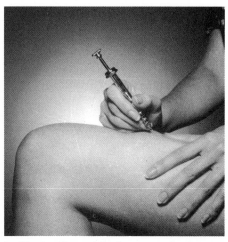

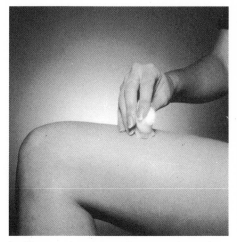

1. Choose the place where you intend to inject your dose of insulin. Make sure area is clean and dry.

2. Pinch skin and fat between the thumb and forefinger of one hand. Hold the syringe by its barrel in the other hand. Quickly inject needle into the skin at an angle of between 45 and 90°.

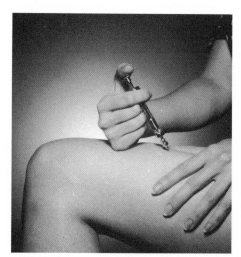

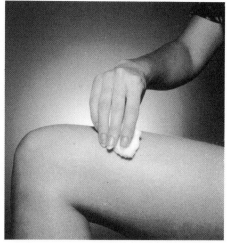

3. Pull back plunger a little and make sure no blood appears in syringe. If there is blood, *don't inject* as it means the needle is in a blood vessel. Withdraw needle and inject in another place. If there's no blood in syringe, press plunger down quickly to inject all the insulin.

4. Quickly pull needle from skin and press on the injection site with cotton wool to prevent any insulin seeping out. Wash out syringe and needle in industrial methylated spirit and store in spirit-proof case provided.

47

Where to inject insulin

The following is a suggested rotation plan for injecting insulin – always check rotation with your doctor first. You should never skip randomly from one part of the body to another; and injections in the same part of the body ought to be spaced about 1 to 1½ in (25 to 38 mm) apart.

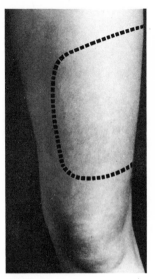

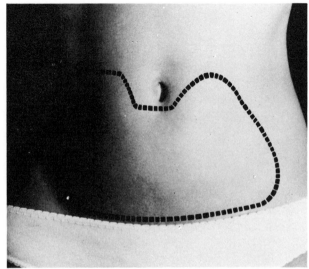

Week 1 Inject the other thigh in **Week 2**.

Week 3

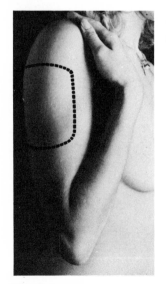

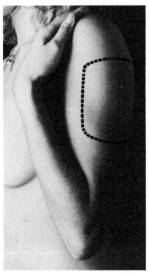

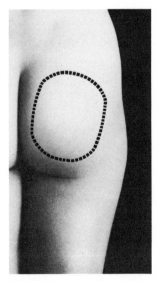

Week 4

Week 5

Week 6 Inject the other buttock in **Week 7**.

Syringes and needles

In North America, Australia and South Africa, most diabetics use disposable syringes and needles—the insulin syringe is marked with 100 graduations to the ml (50 to the $\frac{1}{2}$ ml). Draw up 1 mark per 1 unit. Many syringes come complete with a fused, micro-fine needle 27G$\frac{1}{2}$in.

In Britain many diabetics still use glass insulin syringes, often with disposable needles. The syringe and needle should be kept in industrial methylated spirit in a special carrying case. Change the spirit in the case once a week.

At the time of going to press, U40 and U80 insulins are still used. It is expected to change to U100 insulin shortly. The syringes currently in use are graduated with 20 divisions to the ml (for historical reasons, as they were used with 20 units per ml insulin).

Until the introduction of U100 insulin, the most commonly used insulin in Britain has been 80 units per ml. Patients using 40 units per ml insulin have to divide the number of units by two to give the required number of marks on the syringe. Patients using 80 units per ml insulin have to divide the number of units by four to give the required number of marks on the syringe.

In other European countries 40 units per ml insulin is most commonly used. Most of their syringes have 40 divisions per ml so that 1 unit corresponds to 1 mark.

Mixing two types of insulin in the same syringe

About half my patients who need insulin take a mixture of fast-acting and slow-acting insulin in the morning. This mixture of two types of insulin in the same syringe helps us control their blood sugar better. Often I use a mixture of regular (soluble) and NPH (Isophane) insulins. For a total dose of 32 units a typical mix would be eight units of regular and 24 units of NPH (Isophane). Either type may be drawn into the syringe first but you should always withdraw the insulin from the bottles in the same order to avoid an error in dosage.

1. Mix both bottles of insulin by rolling them in your hands and then clean the tops of the bottles with an alcohol-based cleansing solution.
2. Inject air into one bottle equal to the number of units of insulin to be taken from that bottle. Pull the needle out of the bottle *without* removing any insulin at this time; for example, inject 24 units of air into the NPH (Isophane) insulin bottle.
3. Inject air into the second bottle equal to the number of units to be taken from that bottle. With the needle still in place turn the bottle

49

upside down. Withdraw the number of units needed from the second bottle and check carefully for air bubbles. For example, inject eight units of air into the regular insulin bottle and then withdraw eight units of regular (soluble) insulin.

4. Reinsert the needle into the first bottle and withdraw the number of units needed to make the total dose of the mixture. For example, insert the needle into the NPH (Isophane) insulin bottle and withdraw 24 units of insulin so that your syringe now has a total of 32 units of insulin.

5. Inject the insulin as described.

Do's and don'ts for insulin users

Do

1. Make sure that you have the exact type of insulin that your doctor prescribed.
2. Use the type of syringe that your doctor recommends.
3. Measure your insulin dose carefully.
4. Inject insulin deep under the skin, pointing the needle straight down.
5. Rotate your injection sites so that you do not use the same places all the time.
6. Mix different insulin in the same order each time if you take a mixture of insulins.
7. Keep your current insulin bottle in a cool place such as a cabinet and extra bottles in the refrigerator.
8. Take your insulin at the same time every day.
9. Eat your meals and snacks on time.
10. Wear diabetic identification.
11. Always carry some form of fast-acting sugar with you.
12. Contact your doctor if you have any doubts about your use of insulin.

Don't

1. Use insulin after the expiration date printed on the label.
2. Change the type or brand of insulin unless your doctor tells you to.
3. Shake your bottle of insulin vigorously, as the bubbles prevent you from receiving the proper dose.
4. Use insulin that has lumps, clumps, aggregation or is congealing. (*Note* – all longer-acting insulins are cloudy after mixing.)
5. Change the type of syringe you use, especially if you take a mixture

of insulins.
6. Take other medicines unless you discuss them with your doctor.
7. Omit insulin unless your doctor tells you to.
8. Change the dose of insulin unless previously discussed with your doctor.
9. Inject insulin into your legs before heavy exercise such as running, cycling or swimming.

Side-effects of insulin injections

As well as the insulin reactions already mentioned the other side-effects that can be caused by insulin injections are allergic reactions, insulin antibodies and changes in the fatty tissue.

Allergic reactions   There are two types of allergic reactions. First, a reaction where the actual injection is being given is redness, swelling and itchiness which develops shortly after an insulin injection. This may occur if the injection is not done properly, if the skin is sensitive to the cleansing solution (this occurs less often when 91 per cent isopropyl alcohol is used, which is not available outside North America), or if the patient is allergic to the insulin. If you have this problem you should contact your doctor. Second, a generalized allergy to insulin is rare, but these type of allergic reactions can be very serious. Allergic reactions are now less common than they used to be since the introduction of highly purified insulins.

Most of my patients with a generalized allergy have developed a skin rash on their arms, legs and chest within minutes to hours after their insulin injection. In addition to the skin rash or hives (small areas of swelling, with redness and itchiness of the skin), some patients develop difficulty in breathing, a rapid pulse, sweating and low blood pressure. All these problems need immediate medical attention.

These allergies are usually due to the type of insulin you are using. Most can be corrected or avoided by using a more highly purified form of pork insulin. The development of these purified insulins has been one of the major advances in the treatment of diabetes and the reduction of these allergic reactions.

Insulin antibodies   These develop in most patients treated with insulin, and are also related to the type of insulin used. Most insulins are extracted from cows', or pigs' pancreases. When a non-human insulin is injected the body develops a protective response. Antibodies are proteins in our blood which protect us against foreign materials such as germs. For example, our antibodies against measles and mumps viruses prevent us from developing these diseases again.

Not surprisingly most people who take insulin develop antibodies against beef or pork insulin. These antibodies do not usually cause any problems and most diabetics are not even aware of them in their blood. But in rare instances, very high levels of antibodies may require the use of very large doses of insulin. When a lean person must take over 200 units of insulin a day for a week or longer to control their blood sugar, he or she has insulin resistance. This can usually be treated and corrected with a more highly purified form of pork insulin.

Changes in fatty tissue   With repeated insulin injections some diabetics develop changes in the fatty tissue called the subcutaneous fat, which lies just under their skin. Some people develop hollows or sunken areas over their thighs and other places where insulin has been injected and caused a loss of fatty tissue. This is known as lipoatrophy. Others can develop an excessive accumulation of fat known as hypertrophy, usually caused by using the same areas for injections too frequently. To get rid of hypertrophy the overused areas should be avoided as injection sites for several months. If your doctor gets you to try a more highly purified insulin, this should help you to avoid lipoatrophy. He will give you further advice about how to decrease the atrophy.

Do you need insulin?

In my experience in the United States some adults who take insulin do not absolutely need to. Some patients, though, do require insulin and will need it for the rest of their lives. You will probably always need insulin if: you were started on it before you were thirty years old; you are very lean or skinny and take over 30 units of insulin a day; if you are very lean and exercise a great deal (for example, run 15 miles (24 km) a week or briskly walk 3 miles (5 km) a day) and take over 20 units a day. On the other hand, if you are overweight and not very active you may, with your doctor's help with exercise and losing weight, be able to gradually reduce your insulin dose. (You are overweight if you would have to lose over 20 lb (9 kg), to be very lean.) With a suitable diet, such as the high fiber diets which will be explained in chapter eight, you may even be able to stop your insulin injections. Under no circumstances should you ever attempt to come off insulin except under your doctor's supervision.

RIGHT: It is very important for diabetic shift-workers to plan a convenient schedule with their doctors.

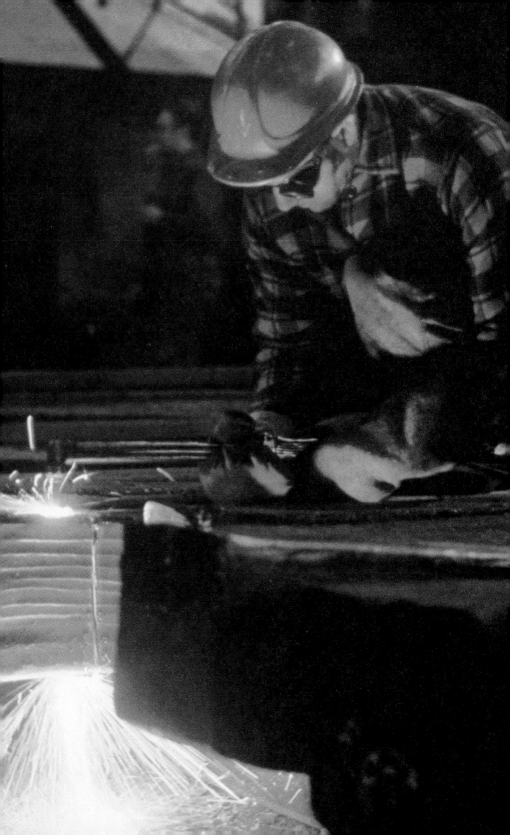

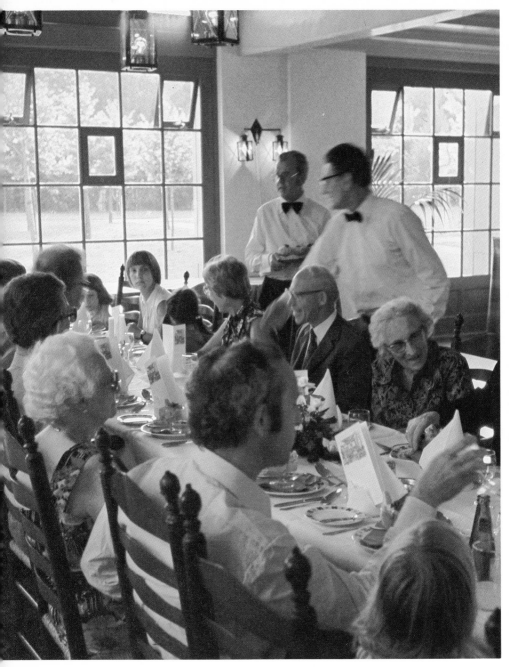

ABOVE: With some ingenuity and tact you can still follow your diet eating out in most restaurants.

RIGHT: When you're invited out for dinner, give your hostess some simple guidelines about your diet.

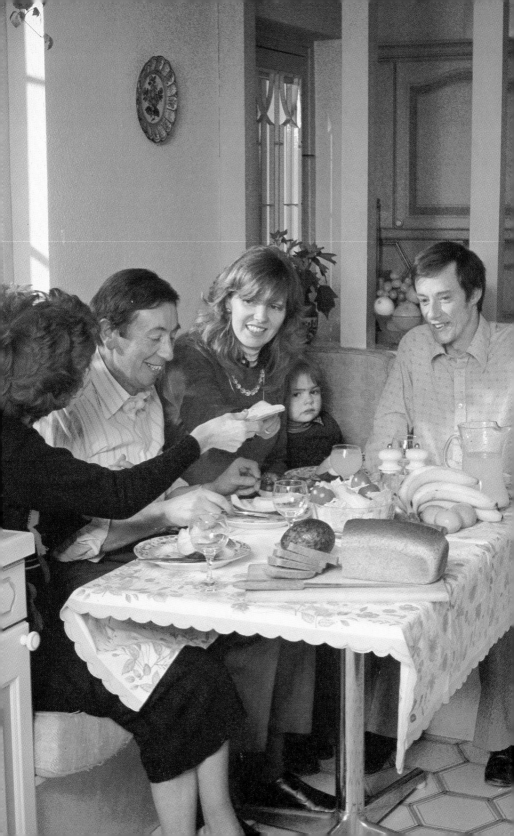

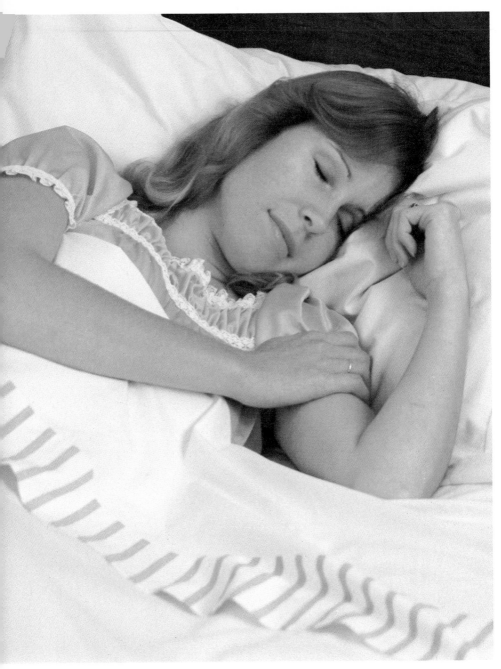

ABOVE: If you get the flu you must try to take your usual insulin dose and carbohydrates, and test frequently.

RIGHT: Your diabetes shouldn't prevent you from getting married.

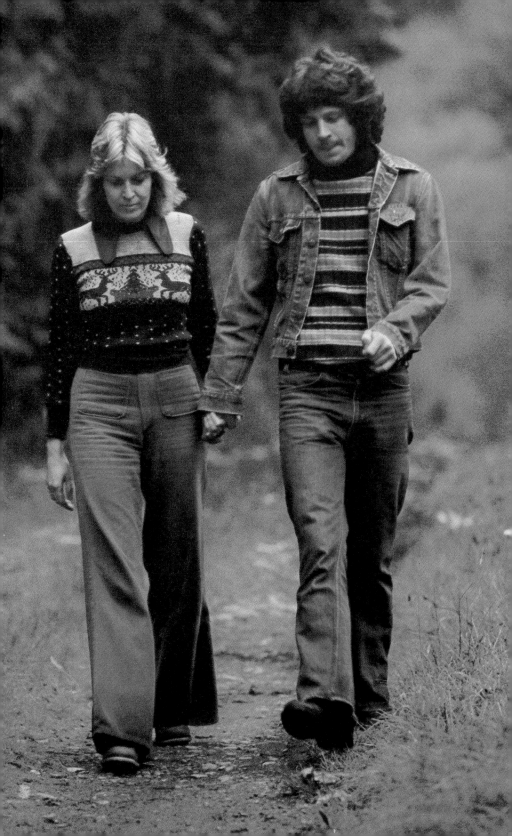

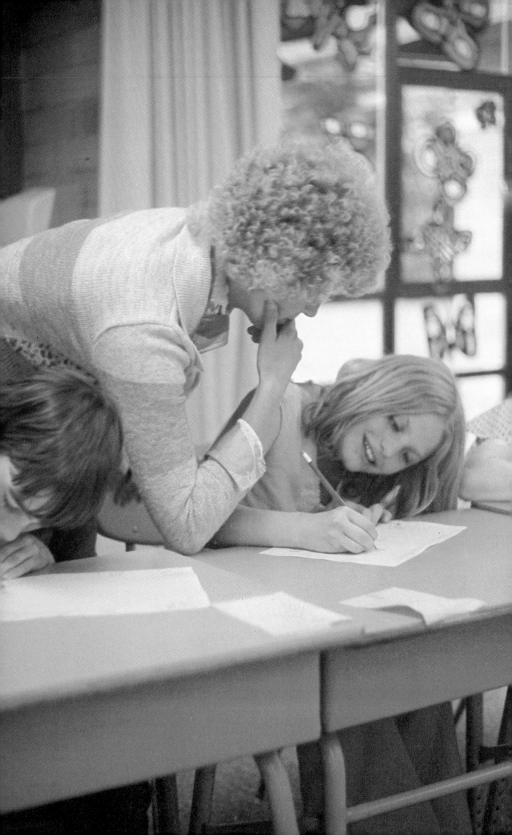

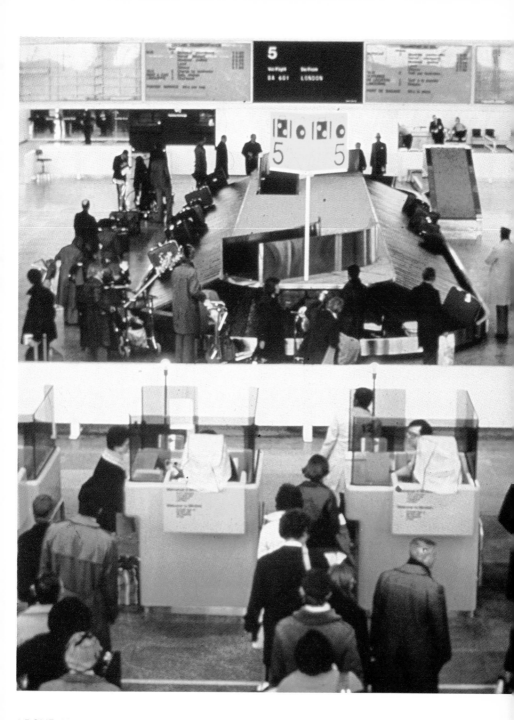

ABOVE: If you take sensible precautions you needn't worry about travelling.
LEFT: Your teacher needs to know that you are diabetic and take insulin.

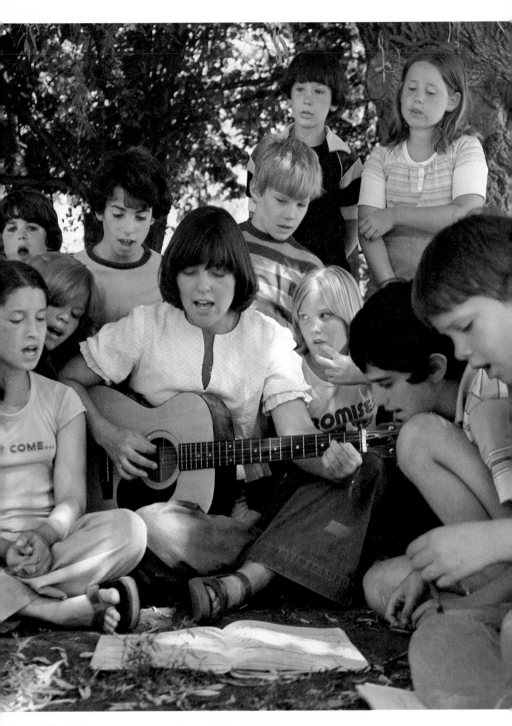

Diabetic camps are great fun and they'll help you.

Antidiabetes pills

Insulin can certainly work miracles and has restored life to millions of diabetics. However, if you do not absolutely need insulin, I think that you are better off with diet treatment, exercise, and antidiabetes pills, if required. Of course any disadvantages associated with taking insulin are minor compared to the advantages of good health that your insulin gives you if you are dependent on it.

So if you can control your blood sugar to your own and your doctor's satisfaction by closely following a diet, taking regular exercise and taking oral antidiabetes pills, I would encourage you to do so. These pills, however, are controversial. You will have to discuss this question with your own doctor.

The use of antidiabetes pills

When your diabetes is almost controlled by diet alone, pills may help you – if your blood sugar has hovered around 200 mg per 100 ml (11 mmol per liter) for months. However, if you need insulin, the pills will not work for you. If you are lean, very active and take over 30 units of insulin per day, it is unlikely that you'll be able to take pills instead of insulin injections. If you are lean and your fasting blood sugar has been above 300 mg per 100 ml (17 mmol per liter) on tests, you probably also need insulin. If you are more than 50 lb (23 kg) overweight, the pills probably wouldn't lower your blood sugar, and you would still need to lose weight. Your doctor must decide for you.

Antidiabetes pills are also called oral hypoglycemic agents, because they lower the blood sugar. They are not a form of oral insulin. The most widely used pills are sulfonylureas which lower the blood sugar by working in two ways. First, they help the pancreas release enough insulin to normalize your blood sugar. Second, they help insulin do its job throughout the body; they make various cells more sensitive to the effects of insulin, so they permit inadequate amounts of insulin to do an adequate job. Other hypoglycemic pills called biguanides are also used, but I will not discuss their effects here.

Antidiabetic pills work very well in the following cases. When lean adults develop a mild form of diabetes and have fasting blood sugars below 200 mg per 100 ml (11 mmol per liter) on our high-fiber maintenance diet, they do very well with small doses of antidiabetes pills. We have stopped insulin treatment for a number of lean patients who closely follow our hospital-controlled high-fiber diets; some of these patients manage to achieve good control with very small doses of pills. We have also taken some obese patients off insulin after they have lost weight, using high-fiber diets and pills to control their blood sugar.

If my patients are overweight and have high blood sugars, they must lose weight. If they are following their diet and losing weight, I sometimes use the pills to lower their blood sugar, but not if they are not losing weight. Sometimes I have to use insulin to treat diabetics who are very overweight.

Two recent patients of mine illustrate how I decide to use the antidiabetes pills.

Juan was a twenty-four year-old dental student. He came to me with all the hallmarks of diabetes and a blood sugar of 312 mg per 100 ml (17 mmol per liter). As he was lean and a jogger, diet was our major hope for him. He went on our high-fiber diet and followed it religiously. Over the next six weeks his blood sugar dropped to 153 mg per 100 ml (8½ mmol per liter), hovering just above our goal of 150 mg per 100 ml (8 mmol per liter). Juan was following the diet and running 20 miles (32 km) per week. To obtain good control we had to start either insulin or the antidiabetes pills; as he had studied pharmacology and understood how drugs work and their side-effects, he wanted to try the pills. I started him on a small dose and his next blood sugar was 106 mg per 100 ml (6 mmol per liter). On small doses of the antidiabetes pills all his blood sugars have been below 110 mg per 100 ml (6 mmol per liter) for the last eighteen months. He feels great and has absolutely no tell-tale symptoms or features of diabetes.

Raymond, a forty-eight year-old carpenter, was a more difficult challenge for our team. He was overweight and came into the hospital taking 40 units of insulin a day. With our high-fiber diet, exercise, and weight loss we were able to stop insulin after three weeks of vigorous treatment. He went home on neither insulin nor pill therapy with blood sugars averaging 140 mg per 100 ml (8 mmol per liter). He followed the diet closely, continued to lose weight and exercised fairly well, but his blood sugar climbed above 200 mg per 100 ml (11 mmol per liter). We had two choices – insulin again or the pills – and mutually we decided to give the pills a short trial. With a moderate dose his blood sugar dropped to less than 150 mg per 100 ml (8 mmol per liter) and he continues to feel well.

Getting off the pills
The only way to get off the pills is to follow a diet, under your doctor's supervision. As long as you follow your diet, you will have good blood sugar reports and your doctor will probably lower your dose – before very long you will be on a small dose of pills and he may feel that you can stop

them altogether.

Side-effects of oral antidiabetes pills
The following side-effects are rare but require prompt medical attention: dark (cola-colored) urine, unusual tiredness, fever and sore throat, unusual bleeding or bruising, or yellow color in the eyes. The following side-effects are more common, they usually disappear after your body adjusts to the medicine, and may not require medical attention unless they are persistent or become a nuisance: diarrhea, nausea, heartburn, stomach discomfort, loss of appetite, or headache.

Skin rashes are less common and skin allergy to the sun may sometimes develop. In my own experience in treating over 500 patients with these drugs, I have only seen side-effects which required stopping the drug in less than a dozen patients.

Oral drugs and heart attacks
Several of my patients have asked me about the report which suggested that one of the oral antidiabetes pills may cause heart attacks. A study called the University Group Diabetes Program (UGDP) compared different treatments for diabetes, including one of the oral drugs (tolbutamide). The results of this study suggest that these drugs might increase the likelihood of deaths from heart attacks. Personally, I have serious reservations about the conclusions drawn from the UGDP study, particularly as other subsequent studies have disagreed with them. This argument has raged since 1970 and is still not settled. Currently, I use the oral drugs in the way described because I think their benefits outweigh their risks for carefully selected patients.

4 COPING WITH DIABETES IN EVERYDAY LIFE

Having dealt with the basic overall control of diabetes, I want in this chapter to answer some of the most common questions my patients ask me about diabetes in everyday life.

Eating out

Can I follow my diet in a restaurant?
If you know which foods you should eat, the serving sizes and how to make substitutions, you can confidently walk into any restaurant. Some people carry small cards in their packets or purse, one set of cards listing food groups or exchanges (see chapter nine), the other, the food choices you have for each meal.

Ask your waitress about portion sizes, how the food is cooked and the ingredients in the menu item, telling her that you are a diabetic and want to avoid hidden sugars and fats. She may advise the chef to 'go easy on the fats'. The restaurant may have skimmed milk, margarine or other items that are not listed on the menu. Don't be afraid to ask questions. With a little ingenuity and tact you can eat well and still follow your diet in most cases.

What are the main problems with restaurant foods?
Most chefs use more fats, oils, sugar and salt than you do at home. In my opinion, fats are the biggest problem for the diabetic. Almost all vegetables served in restaurants are cooked with generous amounts of fat (such as butter). Chicken salads, potato salads and bean salads are often generously laced with dressings. Ask the waitress to serve salad dressings, mayonnaise, butter, margarine, and sour cream separately as a side dish. Ask for dry toast and add your own margarine, if required. If you are having grilled or broiled fish or meat, check that they are grilled or broiled without a lot of fatty cooking oil. Items such as stewed tomatoes may have excessive sugar, and homemade breads often have generous amounts of honey or sugar as well as shortening. As the chef has probably already used salt liberally, you should only add it sparingly; you also may want to take your own sugar substitutes.

What can I order in restaurants?

Appetizers   Low-calorie vegetables such as radishes, celery, carrots and dill (cucumber) pickles; consommé, clear chicken or beef broth, tomato or vegetable juices, or vegetable soups.

Breads   Plain rolls, crackers, melba toast or bread sticks.

Salads   Green vegetable salads with lemon juice or vinegar. Low-calorie dressings are not usually available, so some of my patients carry their own with them in small plastic containers. If you have fat allowances available in your diet (see chapter nine), you can ask for the dressings to be served separately and allow one fat exchange for every tablespoon of dressing you take.

Sandwiches   Based on your bread allowances (see chapter nine) you can select either open (one-slice), regular (two-slice), or club (three-slice) sandwiches. Turkey, sliced chicken, cheese, lean beef or ham are acceptable fillings. Ask for the bread not to be buttered and any dressings (such as mayonnaise) to be served separately. Filleted fish sandwiches are available at some fast food restaurants; ask for separate sauce or remove it.

Meat dishes   Choose baked, grilled or roasted meat, poultry or fish, and remove all visible fat and skin. Avoid gravies and sauces.

Potatoes   Choose baked, broiled, boiled or mashed potatoes. Consider rice or pasta as an alternative; avoid fried potatoes, butter and sour cream.

Vegetables   Choose baked, broiled, boiled, steamed or stewed vegetables. For most vegetable dishes you should omit one fat exchange. If vegetables are unavailable, substitute a third to a half of a bread exchange.

Fats   As many foods served are cooked with extra fat, you should cut down on the amount of margarine you eat.

Desserts   Ask for fresh fruits, or unsweetened canned fruits.

What should I do when a friend invites me home for dinner?
Your friend probably knows that you are diabetic and will want to know what your special needs are. If not, tell your friend that you have diabetes but it does not create a problem; he or she will appreciate knowing these

things. First, that you prefer fresh fruit or unsweetened canned fruit for dessert. Second, that you usually have a green vegetable with your meal; corn, lima and butter beans, and potatoes are starchy items which are considered like breads on your diet instead of vegetables (see chapters six and seven). Third, that you eat only moderate-sized portions of most foods. You can please your hostess or host by praising the food and she or he will not be upset that you eat reasonably little of it.

What do I do when dinner will be served after my regular mealtime?
Possibly you can eat your bedtime snack at 6 pm or your usual mealtime, and then substitute your dinner for your snack. If you are on insulin, you will certainly need to eat something at your regular mealtime. Avoid drinking too much alcohol before this social dinner, or if you do drink some, make sure you eat your snack first. A diabetic, more than anyone else, has to avoid drinking alcohol on an empty stomach as this lowers the blood sugar.

Can I eat cake at weddings and birthday parties?
There are parties and special occasions all the time. Unfortunately, some diabetics are reformed 'sweetaholics'; one piece of cake may send them on a sugar binge. If you have this tendency, you should resist cake at *every* occasion. Provided you are usually able to keep your sweet tooth under control, it is reasonable to have a small square of cake on these very special occasions, even though you are diabetic. You can always remove most of the icing before eating the cake.

Travel
Can a person with diabetes still travel?
After you have mastered the techniques for insulin injections and learned your meal patterns you should certainly be able to travel. You can obtain inexpensive travel kits from many drug stores or pharmacies, but first:

1. Discuss your trip with your doctor before you leave.
2. Ask your doctor to give you a written statement about what medicines and supplies you need. This will get you through customs much easier if you travel abroad.
3. Take along a generous amount of insulin and syringes. In other countries or even other towns your type of insulin or syringe may not be available.
4. Always carry sugar *on your person* to treat low blood sugars. You may not be able to get to the overhead rack or your overnight case if you are developing an insulin reaction.

Your daily schedule

Will I be on a rigid schedule for the rest of my life? I take insulin and my doctor tells me to eat at 6 pm every evening. Also, my diet calls for 120 g (4 oz) of meat each evening. Will I ever be able to alter this program?

A practical program for controlling diabetes must have flexibility, as well as consistency and predictability. However, you are clearly not in total control of your schedule and variations will occur. Furthermore, after you have gained control of your diabetes you will want some flexibility. I am reminded of a movie where a boy captures a beautiful wild stallion, which was totally out of control and difficult to keep in captivity. Slowly the boy gained control and was eventually able to ride the stallion, which became very tame and was free to roam the pastureland without being tied up. Your diabetes, like the stallion, must be completely tamed or controlled. This may require an initial period of discipline, patience, and even rigidity, but after you can control your diabetes and predict its behavior, then you have freedom. You can slowly modify your program to allow a virtually normal lifestyle.

You and your body

How can I find a doctor to treat my diabetes?

If you have recently moved, the following suggestions may be useful in locating a doctor who has a special interest in patients with diabetes. Before moving, ask your doctor whom he recommends in your new neighborhood. Telephone the local diabetes association in your new area, or check with your regional or national association. They will know of doctors who have special interests in diabetes (called endocrinologists or diabetologists). In the United States, the local medical association may be able to tell you of diabetes or internal medicine specialists who have a special interest in treating the disease. In the United States your local library may have a copy of *The Directory of Medical Specialists* which lists specialists in diabetes and endocrinology. Also try asking your minister, local pharmacist or others established in the community. In the United States and Canada look in the yellow pages of your telephone directory to see if there is a diabetes specialist in your area, or you can find the number of your local branch of the American Diabetes Association or your local county medical association in the white pages of the directory. In Britain and Australia your family doctor will recommend you to a diabetes specialist or clinic if he thinks this is necessary.

If you take insulin or pills for your diabetes, I think it is worth your time and effort to find a doctor who has a special interest in the disease, and he is more likely to give you the advice and encouragement you need.

How often should I see my doctor?
I see my diabetic patients every six weeks to four months depending on the nature of their treatment. If your diabetes is well controlled on diet or oral agents every three or four months is probably sufficient. If you are well controlled and stable on insulin therapy, two to three months is average. If, however, you were having problems with your control, I might want to see you every two to six weeks. At each visit I would obtain a blood sugar measurement, and if your diabetes control was fair to good, I would measure the glycohemoglobin concentration every six to twelve weeks. If you had blood fat abnormalities, I would measure your serum cholesterol every three to six months. Every year I take the following tests for each of my patients: X-rays of heart and lungs (chest X-ray), heart tracing (electrocardiogram), complete blood count (red blood count and white blood count), blood fats (cholesterol and triglycerides), kidney tests (blood urea nitrogen, creatinine and urine protein leakage). Always try to have your eyes tested every year. All my patients see an eye specialist (ophthalmologist) at least once a year. Different doctors, of course, have different philosophies and I have outlined my own practice as an example of what would be considered reasonable by many diabetes specialists.

Testing the urine for sugar
Why should I measure the sugar in my urine?
Your urine tests are the most convenient way for you to monitor your diabetes. Some people measure their own blood sugar four times a day; you may not need to do this. When the blood sugar rises above 180 mg per 100 ml (10 mmol per liter), sugar appears in the urine; below this there is no sugar. With a small amount of sugar, your blood sugar has been slightly above 180 mg per 100 ml (10 mmol per liter), and with a large amount the figure is probably above 300 mg per 100 ml (17 mmol per liter). Thus measuring the sugar in your urine serves as a guide to what your blood sugar is doing.

How often should I test my urine?
If you take insulin you should test your urine for sugar before each meal and at bedtime. Always test urine recently made by your kidney: this is called a 'second-voided' or 'double-voided' urine sample (if it has been in your bladder for several hours it will give you incorrect information). You should empty your bladder completely and discard the first specimen; you then test the second specimen passed 15 to 20 minutes later. Keep a record of all urine test results to show to your doctor.

What is the best method for testing my urine for sugar?
If your diabetes is well controlled and you rarely have glucose in the urine, Tes-Tape® is inexpensive and fairly convenient. Tes-Tape® should be protected from light, moisture and heat and stored in a cool dry place. Most of my patients test their urine with Diastix® (dipsticks) instead of Tes-Tape® as they are very convenient.

What do I do if I leave my insulin at home, it gets mislaid or broken?
You can often obtain insulin and syringes from a pharmacy without a prescription. The statement from your doctor will probably convince the pharmacist to meet your request, but if not, you may need a local doctor (such as the hotel doctor or an emergency room doctor) to write you a prescription. If you explain the situation to the doctor's office staff, they may be able to help you more quickly.

What sort of records do I need to keep?
I ask my patients to keep a daily record of urine tests and insulin doses. They also record body weight, insulin reactions, blood sugars and comments (such as 'dinner in restaurant at 9 pm'). These records are very important, as they give us the information required to change the treatment program. Sometimes the patient increases or decreases the insulin dose based on this information, and sometimes I alter the program. They usually also add important comments about their diet each day.

Should I tell my friends that I have diabetes?
Yes, for three good reasons. First, for your own safety the people around you should know that you may have insulin reactions. They should give you sugar if you get weak or start to act peculiarly. Second, for the sake of friendship: your hostess will not be upset if you refuse her latest pastry; your friends will be more tolerant of mood swings and occasional grumpiness. Be careful, though, never to let your diabetes give you an excuse to be a cranky person. Third, as an example, you should admit that you have diabetes – there are too many 'closet' diabetics.

Diabetes is a common disease, and the community needs to know that there are diabetic people who are doing well at their job and are good citizens. We need to dispel the idea that all diabetics end up with amputations or some other dreadful problem.

Why does my diabetes get out of control when I go on vacations?
When you travel by car, train or plane you may be less active than usual and you change your diet. If meals are delayed, you may have an insulin reaction, so you should always carry some type of readily available sugar. Often your blood sugar tends to be higher. You may need to take more insulin, eat less food or find ways to be more active when you are travelling. As a general rule, I advise patients to maintain their same dose of insulin, use moderation in eating, check their urine sugar closely and to 'burn it off' by exercise.

When travelling by car you can walk half a mile every two hours at rest stops. When travelling by air you can walk up and down the aisles, stand for periods and walk at airports at intermediate stops. Usually these measures will keep you in reasonable control until you reach your destination.

Commonsense and diabetes
What sort of identification should I carry?
In your wallet or purse you should have a card saying something like the one below.

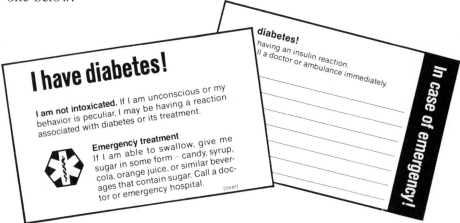

If you take insulin you should wear a bracelet or disc showing that you have diabetes and take insulin. The Medic-Alert bracelets are now used in most countries.

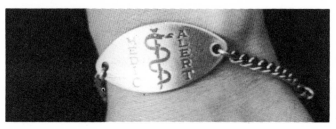

Stress and your diabetes

Can a sinus infection throw my diabetes out of control?
Some of my patients are surprised to learn that even small infections such as a tooth abscess, a sore throat, a large boil or carbuncle, or a sinus infection can cause their blood sugar to shoot up. If you develop a minor infection, you should get treatment; see your dentist or your doctor. In the meantime you should watch your urine readings closely for high sugar or even ketones. You may need to follow your diet especially carefully if you have an infection, and you may need to take extra insulin. Some of my patients take two to five additional units of regular (soluble) insulin once or twice a day till their infection is controlled.

Does emotional stress affect my diabetes?
It certainly can. One of the most vivid examples in my experience was with Maria. This twenty-seven year-old school teacher was 30 weeks pregnant. With two miscarriages behind her she really wanted this baby. I brought her into the hospital to fine-tune her diabetic control, and when her blood sugar was down to 107 mg per 100 ml (6 mmol per liter) I told her she could go home. She called her husband, an unemployed housepainter, but there was no answer. Then another hospital called to tell her that her husband had tried to commit suicide. Although he was all right, she was very upset, and within three hours she was in a mild acidosis. The shock had moved her from excellent control to a near coma state under my very eyes. We were able to get her out of acidosis very quickly and send her home in two days; eight weeks later she had a healthy baby.

Maria's story shows how emotional stress can really mess up your diabetes. If you are a nervous person or feel constant pressure or tension you may need to seek help from your doctor, a psychologist, a comprehensive health center or some other counselling service. They can help you deal with your emotions so that you can better control your diabetes. To reduce stress, anxiety or tension you need to:

1. Analyze the problem and your situation – carefully list everything about which you feel anxious.
2. Develop a plan to reduce the stress. Many popular books are devoted to attacking this problem, but in my experience common-sense is as good as sophisticated techniques. Avoid drugs and alcohol as ways to treat stress and anxiety – they only replace one problem with another.
3. Test your plan and keep working on it – you need to have long-range plans to combat stress and must work persistently at controlling these factors.

Special problems
What should I do if I get the flu?
The three cardinal rules are: first, take your usual dose of insulin; second, test your urine frequently; third, try to eat your usual amount of carbohydrates (sugars and starches). You must take your insulin, the stress of your illness will raise your blood sugar even if you do not eat. Monitoring your urine tests will tell you if you need more insulin. If you are running a reading of 2 per cent sugar and moderate or strong acetone, you should call your doctor, as he may require you to take extra insulin. Eating is very important even if you don't feel hungry; unrefined carbohydrate intake helps to keep the ketones from accumulating in your blood and urine. You should also call your doctor if you have a high temperature, vomit a great deal, or have a persistent bad pain.

During a temporary illness unrelated to diabetes, you need to eat carbohydrates (sugars and starches) and drink plenty of fluids. Don't worry about proteins (meats, cheese and milk) and fats. Try to drink 4 fluid oz ($\frac{1}{2}$ cup) of liquid every one to two hours. Fruit juices, cola drinks (*not* the sugar-free type) and ginger ale, are good sources of carbohydrate. When you are ill you can eat ice-cream, sherbet, Jello® (jelly in Britain) and sweetened custard. Eat food that will agree with you, such as soups, crackers, toast, and fruits – try to eat at least 150 g (5 oz) of carbohydrate per day. Cola drinks have 40 g ($1\frac{1}{2}$ oz) of carbohydrate per 360 ml (12 fluid oz), bread has 15 g ($\frac{1}{2}$ oz) per slice, cereals have 15 g per serving, and fruit has 10 to 15 g per serving.

I am having three teeth pulled in the morning. What should I do about my food and insulin?
Get up early, take your usual dose of insulin and eat your usual breakfast about two hours before your dental appointment. After the visit to the dentist, check your urine for sugar and acetone. If both are strongly positive, you may need extra regular insulin – call your doctor. If the urine sugar test is less than 2 per cent and there is no acetone, you are doing fine. At midday, have your usual amount of carbohydrates as liquids, such as cola, ginger ale or fruit juices. For your snacks and evening meal, make certain that you take in your usual amount of carbohydrates in juices, regular carbohydrate beverages (*not* the sugar-free type), ice cream, Jello® (jelly in Britain) as mentioned above. Check your urine frequently and call your doctor if you have strongly positive tests for sugar and acetone in your urine. The following case history illustrates the potential problems of tooth extraction.

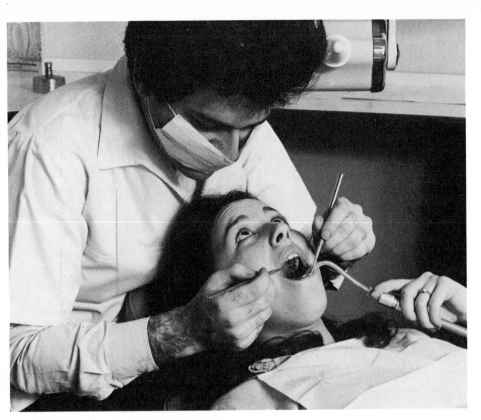

Susan, a twenty-seven year-old secretary, showed that a person can develop ketoacidosis even with plenty of insulin available. Even though she had been diabetic since the age of twelve, she had only been in ketoacidosis once, at fourteen. She came into the hospital to have her remaining teeth extracted. She was not able to eat for three days after surgery. We gave her plenty of insulin but not enough sugar or carbohydrates, so unfortunately she developed a moderate degree of ketoacidosis under my supervision. She improved when given adequate insulin and fluids, and soon after we made certain that she received adequate sugar or carbohydrates.

What should I do if I forget to take my insulin one morning?
Call your doctor! If he is unavailable, the following general guidelines will help. If you discover before noon that you have not taken your morning dose of insulin, take 75 per cent of your dose of slow-acting insulin (NPH Isophane or Lente) and 50 per cent of your dose of fast-acting insulin like regular (soluble). If you discover your error before 4 pm take half your dose of intermediate-acting insulin and no regular (soluble) insulin. Check your urine frequently for sugar and ketones and watch for hypoglycemia.

On the next day, resume taking your usual dose of insulin. Put reminders on your bathroom mirror and refrigerator: 'Take insulin'.

I work night shifts from 11 pm until 7 am, five days a week. When should I take my insulin?
You and your doctor will have to find a schedule that works for you. Most of my patients who work the night shift take two shots of insulin a day, usually about two-thirds of their daily dose in the evening before they go to work, and the remainder after they get home the next morning. On days off, they take about half their daily dose in the morning and about half before the evening meal. Your insulin program will depend on your own work, eating and exercise patterns.

The following case history concerns a night-shift worker.

Tony, a thirty-seven year-old assembly line worker, worked the graveyard shift (from 11 pm to 7 am) Monday to Friday. His diabetes was poorly controlled when he came to see me. He was taking 50 units of NPH (Isophane) at 10 pm from Monday to Friday, and then taking his next injection at 10 am on Sunday – only six doses a week! He went for 36 hours between injections twice weekly (from Friday evening until Sunday morning and from Sunday morning to Monday night). We worked out a better program for him and changed his insulin schedule over the weekend so that he took insulin every 12 hours. This greatly improved his blood sugar control.

Marriage and the family
Should a diabetic get married?
Most young people with diabetes can marry, have healthy children, pursue active careers, and suffer very little disability from their diabetes. If you have had diabetes for less than ten years and have taken good care of it, have no eye or kidney disease, I have no reservations about marriage plans. I think you can maintain the status quo and prevent the development of future problems. You can probably work a full week, have minimal health-related problems, and care for your family. I am optimistic about the future, but I am also realistic about the past. If you have had diabetes for a long time and have not been able to take good care of it, I think you should have a careful medical check-up.

Before making a final decision about marriage, discuss your particular problem first with your future husband or wife. You should get your eyes checked to find out whether you have serious eye disease which threatens your vision; your blood and urine should be carefully examined to determine if you have any other problems such as kidney damage. However, a strong commitment on your part to take care of your diabetes will reduce the chances of these problems getting worse.

Should a diabetic person have children?
A diabetic man should have no problem becoming a father. A diabetic woman whose diabetes is well controlled should have little problem getting pregnant. If you take insulin, becoming a mother may represent a heavier commitment of energy, time and money. Fortunately over 90 per cent of diabetic women today can give birth to healthy babies. Achieving this dramatic increase has required vigorous medical management. You will have to keep your blood sugar normal all the time, perhaps even measuring it at home. You will have to see your doctor almost every week and may need to be in hospital for several weeks. A healthy baby is worth it.

Will my children develop diabetes?
It is very difficult to predict who will develop the disease, as it is inherited through a very complex process. Also, juvenile-type diabetes may result from an unfortunate coincidence – perhaps a viral infection in a child with an inherited tendency for the disease. If you have the juvenile-type, the chances of your child developing this type of diabetes appears to be less than one in ten. At the very worst, if you have identical twins and one develops the juvenile-type, the second twin has only a 50 per cent chance of developing this type of diabetes. If both parents have diabetes, three out of four of their children will eventually develop it, and one of these is likely to have the juvenile-type.

Everyday problems
When should I test my urine for ketones?
Most of my patients check their urine closely for sugar but not for ketones. When someone spills ketones frequently or is subject to acidosis, I have them test their urine routinely with Ketodiastix® which measures sugar and ketones.

Usually I tell my patients taking insulin to check for ketones under the following circumstances. If their urine has 2 per cent or more sugar for two consecutive tests or the blood sugar reading is over 100 mg per 100 ml ($5\frac{1}{2}$ mmol per liter) higher than their usual reading for two consecutive tests; if they have a fever; if they develop nausea or vomit; if they make an error in their insulin dose; if they get injured, or have minor surgery. You can test for ketones (acetone) with Ketostix® and Acetest® tablets which are available in most countries and Ketodiastix® strips in North America. When ketones are present, the strips or tablets turn light or dark purple indicating moderate or large amounts. If you show dark purple you should contact your doctor.

Does it matter where in my body I inject the insulin?
It is *very important* to take your injections in different parts of your body. You should use your legs, stomach and arms (perhaps someone in your family can give you your arm injections). Of course, it is less painful to go to the same place each time – the nerves are deadened and the injections hurt less. But this causes two problems. First, fatty tissue accumulates in the region where you take your injection – check if you have a lump of fatty tissue on your legs. You will not look good in a bathing-suit if these lumps grow too large. Second, your insulin is not absorbed as well from these fatty lumps; on certain days it may be released too rapidly from the lumps and cause a reaction, or too slowly and you will run high sugar all day. In the long run it pays to rotate your injections.

For the younger diabetic
Should I tell my friends that I have diabetes?
Yes, for two reasons. First, if you start acting oddly your friends will know to give you sugar; also, they won't offer you candy unless you need it. Second, your friends will respect you more if you do your share; for example, they may say, 'He's a good ballplayer and doesn't let his diabetes bother him'. The worst thing you can do is try to hide your diabetes – your friends will think you are strange and not know why, and won't understand why the teacher gives you special privileges.

What should my teacher know about my diabetes?
Your teachers, the school nurse (if there is one), and the secretary should know that you have diabetes and take insulin. They should know what an insulin reaction is and how to treat it. They will all want to help you if you and your parents are honest with them. If you do your school work well, your teachers will respect you.

What are diabetic camps?
Most diabetic camps are fun. They were started to encourage lots of activities with good supervision. You can swim, hike, play sports or just do what you want. Doctors and nurses are available if your diabetes gets out of control. You will be camping with about 75 other diabetic young people and will have a lot in common with them. You and the staff and the

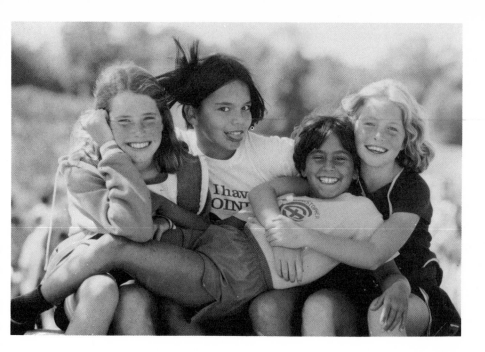

other young people can exchange tips about diabetes. Your parents can obtain further information about diabetic camps by writing to your local or national diabetes association. The diabetes associations in North America, Britain, Australia and most other countries hold diabetic camps.

Sometimes I run around all day and my sugar gets too low. Other days I stay indoors and my sugar gets too high. What can I do?
When you are playing hard, you need extra food. Your mother and your doctor can work out what you should eat. If you are playing a ballgame, eat your entire meal before starting, and take some food to eat during the game – fruits or fruit juices give you energy fast. Be sure to eat something as soon as the game is over. The secret of avoiding low blood sugars is to eat food to replace the calories you burn up; on a less active day you will not need a large snack. Your urine tests may tell you how much to eat. If there is no sugar in the urine, you can eat a large snack; if the glucose test is $\frac{1}{2}$ per cent or more you may need a small snack.

Which method do you recommend for testing young diabetics' urine?
You are more active than adults and your urine tests show a wider range of sugar. I recommend that you use the two-drop or five-drop Clinitest® method for better accuracy. Diastix® are more convenient and are relatively accurate, provided you always remember to wait at least 30 seconds before checking the color of the strip.

5 WHEN DIABETES GETS OUT OF HAND

High blood sugars can be dangerous

You will already have gathered that it isn't healthy to have high blood sugars. The accumulation of sugar in different parts of the body such as your eyes, for example, will start to interfere with their normal working. Also, the body's white blood cells become lazy and don't repel bacteria invasion, so infections are more likely to develop. Good control of blood sugar can certainly prevent most potential problems. Some people may have a tendency to develop eye or kidney trouble just the same and good control may not prevent these problems.

For years the dreaded complications of blindness, amputations and kidney failure were skeletons in the diabetes closet. Parents of diabetic children were especially frightened by these complications, as until recently very little was known about the reasons for them. Medical research has shown that most complications are related to the length of time and severity of the high blood sugars. If you have moderately high blood sugars consistently, say between 250 mg per 100 ml and 350 mg per 100 ml (14 mmol and $19\frac{1}{2}$ mmol per liter), you are more likely to develop tissue damage.

Most diabetics don't develop serious problems; some patients take excellent care of their diabetes for 25, 30 and even 40 years and have absolutely no trouble. Current research suggests that restoring the blood sugar to normal using modern laboratory tests, insulin infusion pumps or multiple insulin shots will prevent most problems. Getting satisfactory blood sugar readings is more difficult for some diabetics than others, but persevering with this is well worth the effort.

Problems that diabetics can face

These are influenced by the age at which they contract diabetes. Kidney disease is a major problem for children who develop diabetes and accounts for 46 per cent of all deaths. In adults kidney failure strikes down only 2 per cent – their major problem is hardening of the arteries. Heart attacks, strokes and gangrene account for 72 per cent of all deaths in adult-type diabetics, but only 33 per cent in the juvenile-type group. Comas are responsible for 5 per cent of deaths in the juvenile-type and only 1 per cent in the adult-type group. Infections lead to loss of life in about 7 per cent of cases in both groups.

Damage to small blood vessels

Capillaries, the very smallest blood vessels known, are most severely affected by poorly controlled diabetes. These tiny blood vessels carry oxygen and nutrients to all the body's cells. When these passages become clogged the cells do not receive adequate oxygen or food. Like gasoline engines our tissues require the proper mixture of oxygen and fuel to run properly.

Persistent high blood sugars weaken the blood vessel walls which become thicker but more porous. Proteins and other constituents of the blood can leak out into the tissues; outpouchings or blisters, known as aneurysms, can develop in the small blood vessel. Damage to these leads to damage of the eyes, the kidneys and other tissues. Some minor damage to the capillaries is usually present in all diabetics except where blood sugar control is exceptionally good.

Kidney trouble

Between 25 and 40 per cent of all people who have had diabetes for over 25 years have problems with their kidneys. The actual position is probably better than this as the statistics include many people whose diabetes had been very badly controlled over a long period. However, with careful control of the blood sugar this might drop to well below 10 per cent. Kidney trouble has the following symptoms:

1. Sticky urine caused by leakage of protein, soon followed by swelling around the ankles, known as edema.
2. A general feeling of fatigue caused by waste products called urea accumulating in the blood. This is known as uremic poisoning.

Each kidney has over a million filtration units called glomeruli, which remove waste products, toxic materials, salts and water from the blood. These substances are then excreted in the urine. Each glomerulus is spherical and completely filled with capillaries, like a hollow rubber ball filled with thin hollow tubes. With every heartbeat the kidneys receive about a quarter of the total blood distributed to the body. Since the two kidneys represent less than 1 per cent of the total body weight they receive a very large share of the blood supplied to the body. In the early stages of diabetes the blood flow to the kidneys increases even further, so these high flow rates may contribute to early damage to the capillaries in the glomeruli.

With consistent very high blood sugars, over a period of a few years, the capillary walls start to leak proteins and other materials as described above (these proteins can be detected in the urine). Also, with high blood sugars the outer walls of the blood vessels grow thicker each year. These glomeruli, like hollow rubber balls, cannot expand in size. So thickening of the capillary walls must compress other hollow tubes, and as a result blood flow is blocked and the glomeruli are damaged. As capillary passages in many glomeruli are closed off, the amount of blood that the kidney is able to filter is reduced. So urea collects in the blood and causes uremic poisoning.

But again this whole process can hopefully be prevented by maintaining a satisfactory blood sugar, and kidney damage if detected early, can even be reversed – the thick gelatinous coat can shrink. For example if small amounts of protein appear in your urine as a result of diabetes, good control could later lead to healing of the capillaries, and the protein leakage would disappear.

If, however, there is substantial damage to the kidneys resulting in large amounts of protein leakage (several grams per day) or uremic poisoning, this may be too severe to be reversible.

Eye disease

Minor damage to the blood vessels to the eye is found in about 70 per cent of people who have had diabetes for at least 25 years. Serious damage which may threaten vision can occur in about a third of this group. Diabetic patients may develop cataracts (cloudiness of the lens) or glaucoma (high pressure in the eyeball). The major concern, though, is damage to the blood vessels of the retina, the back part of the eye. As in the kidney, the small blood vessels may be damaged by chronically high blood sugars, but with good control of the blood sugar and active treatment by an eye specialist, blindness can be prevented in many cases.

The capillaries in the retina tend to develop outpouchings or blisters called microaneurysms. Blood can also leak from damaged capillaries. If blood accumulates over important areas for vision or seeps into the part known as the vitreous chamber, vision may be lost or impaired. A major concern is that the leakage of blood may separate the retina from its supporting structures; this is known as retinal detachment. Fortunately, today all these problems can be corrected or prevented. Vision can even be restored to an eye damaged by hemorrhage.

Good diabetic control is the best way to maintain normal vision by

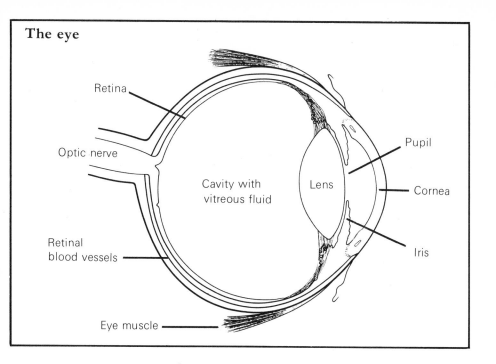

The eye

Retina

Optic nerve

Cavity with vitreous fluid

Lens

Pupil

Cornea

Iris

Retinal blood vessels

Eye muscle

preventing damage or leakage in these capillaries. When the blood vessels are damaged, they decrease the delivery of blood to the retina; new blood vessels are formed to provide additional blood supply, but unfortunately these are very fragile and hemorrhage quite easily.

These problems may be improved or corrected by new techniques such as photocoagulation or laser therapy, techniques which focus a beam of light on a very tiny area of the retina. This beam is so intense that it causes a small burn, which may close off a leaking blood vessel. These techniques act like a magnifying glass focussing the sun rays on a leaf to burn it.

To detect eye disease early, every diabetic should have a complete eye examination at least once a year. By injecting a special dye, eye problems can be discovered early, and laser therapy is very effective in preventing further damage. A detached retina, for instance, can often be reattached to its supporting structures, or, when blood accumulates in the vitreous chamber, it can often be removed.

Nerve damage
At least 65 per cent of diabetics who have had the disease for 25 years or more develop nerve damage, particularly in the legs and feet. This toxic effect on nerves is similar to the effects of high sugars on the lens; the nerves accumulate excessive quantities of sugar and sugar products, leading to nerve swelling and disruption of function. In addition the

excess of sugar prevents the production of a special sugar known as myoinisitol which is important for nerve function. The functions of the nerves to the legs and feet which carry signals to the muscles (motor nerves), and also sensations of feelings and pain (sensory nerves) from the legs, are impaired by high blood sugars.

If your blood sugar has been moderately high for three or four weeks you may have noticed a tired or aching feeling in your legs, or a numbness when you crossed them. Some people develop areas that are very sensitive to touch and even to the pressure of their bed-sheets. Others have prickling 'pins and needles' sensations. All these problems usually clear up within a few weeks after the blood sugar has been brought under satisfactory control. These problems are termed acute or short-term neuropathies.

With longstanding diabetes, other types of neuropathies may develop, and some are not reversible since the chronic toxic effects of high blood sugars has caused irreparable damage to the nerves. In the motor nerves this may lead to muscle weakness and even to a foot drop (the inability to raise the foot), and in the sensory nerves may result in decreased ability to feel pain, heat or touch in the feet.

The autonomic nervous system, a special system of nerves which regulates many automatic functions of the body not under direct voluntary control, may also be damaged by high blood sugars. Emptying of the stomach, sexual functions and blood pressure are controlled by this system. As a result of diabetes, food may not empty properly from the stomach, and there may be diarrhea and loss of bladder control; some men lose the ability to obtain an erection of the penis (impotence). Unfortunately these abnormalities are usually permanent because the toxic effects of high blood sugars has led to nerve damage. However, as some people may improve with good control, I tend to be optimistic with most of my patients.

Foot problems

Because of lack of normal feeling, poor circulation and impaired healing, some diabetics are particularly subject to foot problems. Injuries or infections involving the feet are serious threats to the diabetic, as either may result in loss of the leg or even loss of life. Most of these problems can be avoided by a commonsense approach to taking care of the feet. We estimate that 70 to 80 per cent of amputations caused by gangrene could be avoided if the diabetic had followed the guidelines outlined below. At our hospital we have developed the following 'do's and don'ts' for foot care.

Do

1. Look at your feet daily. Clean minor injuries twice a day with mild soap and water or a mild antiseptic and cover with a sterile dressing. Tell your doctor or nurse if you have sore places that do not heal up. See your doctor at once if you have a break in the skin associated with redness, swelling, drainage or pain. Check closely for fungal infections and report to your doctor if you have cracked, peeling, weeping or itching skin between your toes.
2. Wash your feet daily with mild soap and lukewarm water (40 °C or 104 °F). Test the water temperature with your wrist or elbow. Wash and dry well especially between your toes. Pat or blot your feet dry without rubbing.
3. Treat dry skin with a lanolin-type lotion or cream, baby oil or mineral oil, applying immediately after bathing and rubbing well but gently. Dust with talcum or baby powder.
4. Cut or file your toenails straight across, but *not* too short. Cut the nail even with the end of the toe using a good light after a bath. If you do not see well, ask someone else to do this for you. If you have ingrown toenails, place lambswool or cottonwool under the corner of the nail.
5. Consult your doctor or podiatrist or chiropodist (foot doctor) if you have corns, callouses, ingrown toenails or need special arch support.
6. If your toes overlap, separate them with lambswool, but this must not encircle the toes as it is liable to shrink and cut into the skin.
7. Wear clean socks or stockings every day. Be certain that the socks fit properly and avoid holes and darns.
8. Wear good-fitting lace-up shoes made from soft leather. Be certain that your shoes are neither too tight nor too loose. Avoid slippers or shoes with an open toe. Break in new shoes slowly. Keep shoes in good repair and check the inside often for sharp tacks.

Don't

1. Go barefoot even on the beach.
2. Injure your toes, feet or legs if possible.
3. Put hot water bottles or heating pads on feet or legs.
4. Wear tight socks or garters.
5. Cross your legs with pressure on the back of the knee.
6. Use iodine, betadine, corn cures, bleach, lysol, carbolic acid or any other strong chemicals on your feet.
7. Put adhesive strapping directly over a wound.
8. Try to remove corns, callouses or ingrown toenails.

9. Walk on a sore foot.
10. Smoke, as it interferes with circulation to your feet.
11. Delay medical care when you have a foot problem.

Remember that your feet are priceless and they need special care so that they can serve you well.

It is essential that diabetics understand that their sense of feeling of pain or heat or cold may be dulled, and that their circulation may be less efficient than in a non-diabetic of similar age.

Hardening of the arteries

This condition can cause heart attack and stroke in the adult population at large. A million Americans die from heart disease and stroke each year. We still don't know exactly what makes this problem so common in North America, Europe, Australasia and most other developed parts of the world. What is clear is that there are three major risk factors – high blood fat levels, high blood pressure and cigarette smoking. Diabetics often have high blood cholesterol levels, and kidney damage can cause a greater risk of high blood pressure.

Hardening of the arteries is known as arteriosclerosis. Fatty deposits containing cholesterol build up in the walls of the arteries. Over the years they cause a gradual blocking of the passage through the arteries restricting the free flow of blood. Eventually this blockage may cause heart attack or stroke.

The platelets (or thrombocytes) in the blood help clotting and healing of damaged blood vessels. Platelets can also cause formation of small plaques or bumps that interfere with the normal ability of the artery wall to push out cholesterol which accumulates below the plaque. In diabetics the platelets seem to stick together more easily, and may lead to more silting up of the arteries than in non-diabetics.

Being overweight also increases the likelihood of arterial disease and heart attack. There is growing evidence that a reasonable amount of exercise can help reduce hardening of the arteries.

Preventing hardening of the arteries

Heart attacks which result from hardening of the arteries have only become common during the twentieth century with increasing industrialization. Evidence from hundreds of animal experiment studies shows that hardening of the arteries can be produced by feeding cholesterol and animal fat. Recent studies using special X-rays have shown that reducing blood fats in people with high levels of cholesterol and triglycerides caused a reversal of their arteriosclerosis. Your doctors can measure your blood cholesterol level, which ideally should be kept within the healthy range below 180 mg per 100 ml (10 mmol per liter).

Three dietary factors seem to affect cholesterol levels in the blood, so to lower the level of cholesterol in your blood you should:

1. Eat less cholesterol which is most commonly found in egg yolks, dairy products, organ meats such as heart, liver, kidney and brains, shrimp, beef, pork, veal and lamb.

2. Restrict total fat intake to less than 30 per cent of calories if you have high blood cholesterols. Saturated animal fats sustain the blood cholesterol, whereas unsaturated vegetable fats lower it. As you limit your meat intake to avoid cholesterol, you automatically lower your intake of saturated fats. When you obtain protein from plant sources you are automatically substituting unsaturated fats for saturated fats.

3. Eat certain type of fibers which lower the blood cholesterol level. Oat bran and dried beans contain these fibers. We give our patients about 50 g ($1\frac{1}{2}$ oz) of oat bran per day (one bowl of cereal and four oat bran muffins). Unfortunately oat bran is not yet commercially available outside North America. By eating oatmeal daily, and dried beans (such as kidney, pinto, navy and haricot beans) several times a week, you can maintain a lower blood cholesterol level.

Your diet not only has an important place in preventing hardening of the arteries but also in treating your diabetes. We have found that the same dietary principles apply both to diabetics and to patients with hardening of the arteries. A prudent diet, generous in unrefined starchy foods and restricted in fat and cholesterol, is of benefit to almost everyone.

6 YOUR KEY TO A HEALTHY DIET

A new approach to diabetic diets

In chapter two I said that diet is the first of the three legs enabling you to control your diabetes. This vital factor has long been ignored by many doctors. They previously prescribed a diet for their diabetic patients with a lot of fat and virtually no carbohydrates like bread and potatoes – the exact opposite of what we now recommend!

The calories and elements that make up your daily diet are all carefully graded in our diabetic diet program. The main nutrients in food are carbohydrates, proteins, fats, and small amounts of vitamins and minerals.

What we need from our diet

Carbohydrates   These provide us with important sources for our daily energy and are found mainly in plant foods. There are two different kinds of carbohydrate – sugars and starches. Fruit and green vegetables provide sugars known as simple carbohydrates. Cereal grains such as wheat, oats, barley and rice, potatoes and dried beans are all rich in starches known as complex carbohydrates. This group will help you control your diabetes better and are emphasized in our program. They are also surprisingly low in calories as explained below.

Try to avoid eating added table sugar (sucrose) and sugary foods as much as you can. They contain a lot of 'empty' calories and no vitamins or minerals, and cause weight gain which is bad for most adults, but especially for diabetics. Many people recommend honey instead of sugar, but I have not found that it provides any particular advantage for diabetic patients.

Proteins   These come from meats, poultry, fish, dairy products and, to a lesser extent, from plant foods. Young people need more protein while they are still growing. For adults, protein is used to repair and replace damaged body tissue.

All adults should receive at least 45 g (1½ oz) of protein per day. This could be provided by eating just 90 g (3 oz) of chicken, one glass of milk and half a cup of lima or butter beans (90 g/3 oz). Of course, most western people eat far more protein than this. Unlike fats, proteins do not affect blood sugar levels.

Fats   Fats are found in most animal and plant foods. But whereas most vegetables and fruits contain only trace amounts of fats, most meats have generous amounts of saturated fats, and eating these may keep your blood cholesterol at unhealthily high levels. Vegetable fats though, such as corn oil, are high in unsaturated fats and will lower your blood cholesterol.

As a diabetic, you should avoid fat intake whenever possible. Fats block the action of insulin in the blood whether this is produced naturally in your pancreas or injected. Our bodies only require a minimum of 5 g of fat a day. Most Americans eat ten or twenty times that.

I recommend that you get only 20 to 25 per cent of your total daily calories from fat, which is about 35 to 50 g (1 to 2 oz) of fat a day; 180 g (6 oz) of roast beef with 25 per cent of fat by weight has a total of about 45 g ($1\frac{1}{2}$ oz) of fat. This is nine times our minimum requirement and is equal to our entire daily needs of fat on a 2000 calorie diet. When our patients restrict their intake of fats and cholesterol their insulin needs decline and their blood fats are lower.

With our diet program, many of my patients with less severe diabetes can stay off insulin by limiting their fat intake provided they also significantly increase the amount of fiber-rich food they eat. They trim off all the visible fat from meat, remove the skin from poultry, and eat bread and potatoes without butter, margarine or sour cream. So it is fats and oils that are the enemies of good diabetic control.

Vitamins   In basic chemistry, substances are either organic (derived from living things such as animals or plants) or inorganic (minerals from non-living sources). Vitamins are organic substances which our bodies require in small amounts to function properly. Our bodies can't produce adequate quantities of most vitamins and so we need to rely on our foods to provide them. Human beings need 13 or 14 different vitamins from a wide variety of both animal and plant sources – such as green vegetables, grains and fruits, meat, fish and poultry. If you eat these, you are probably getting naturally a generous supply of these essential vitamins.

Minerals   We need seven major minerals for the structure of our bodies and to keep them working properly: sodium chloride (salt), potassium, calcium, phosphorus, magnesium and sulfur. These are obtained from a wide range of vegetable and animal foods. The remaining minerals are called trace minerals – iron and iodine, for instance – because we only get or need small or trace amounts from our diets. The other trace minerals include lead and mercury and are called contaminants because they are not required for body functions. In fact, excessive intakes can cause very serious damage to the body – lead poisoning which can cause nerve damage is a good example.

Fiber   Although not a nutrient, fiber derived from plant foods and sometimes known as roughage is now recognized by most doctors and scientists as vital for everyone's diet, increasing bulk in our diet without adding calories. Fiber forms the skeleton of all plants, and also provides their protective outer coating of shell or husk.

Until very recently the importance of fiber in our diet was largely ignored by doctors and nutritionists. Foods naturally richest in fiber are the starchy carbohydrates. The dry weight of some cereal grains contain up to 50 per cent fiber; wheat kernels for example are rich in fiber, but when they get milled into flour, the modern mills strip away the kernels' outer covering which is richest in fiber.

When high-fiber foods are less heavily processed they contain more vitamins and minerals. Usually they need more chewing and must be eaten more slowly. This is much healthier than gobbling food down quickly.

Accurate tests have recently been devised by scientists to measure the fiber content of foods. These are shown in the *Guide to fiber in foods* section in chapter nine (page 141). The fiber content of many of these foods had not been measured before, and had to be measured specially in my laboratory. Fiber helps the movement of food along the gut. Scientists have found that some parts of fiber absorb water in the small intestine like gelatin powder or Jello® (jelly in Britain), retaining sugars and starches and slowing down their absorption in the body. It also binds other substances such as vitamins, minerals and bile acids. If the bile acids are retained by fiber, there is growing evidence that less cholesterol is absorbed by the body.

With enough fiber, bowel movements will be larger and softer. No laxatives would be necessary if everyone ate enough fiber, and piles or hemorrhoids would be much less of a problem. There is also growing evidence that fiber in the diet may protect against diabetes, heart attacks, strokes and colon cancer, and prevent obesity. Dr Denis Burkitt and Dr Hugh Trowell have made scientific studies comparing the occurrence of these and other diseases in North America and other developed countries with their relative occurrence in parts of the world such as tribal Africa.

Their conclusions suggest that a high-fiber diet would protect against these diseases. A companion volume to this book (*Don't Forget Fibre in Your Diet*) has been written by Dr Burkitt describing this fascinating story for the general reader.

My dietary recommendations in chapter nine are based on treating about 200 patients for up to six years on high-fiber programs. They were all able to control their blood sugar better, and under careful medical supervision most of them were also able to reduce their insulin requirements, and significantly reduce their blood fat levels. We also found these diets useful for weight loss, where necessary, because they are filling but also low in calories.

By introducing a variety of interestingly prepared foods, patients found no problem in increasing their fiber daily intake to between 40 and 60 g ($1\frac{1}{2}$ and 2 oz) of fiber. The diet provides fiber from a variety of natural foods, and as long as it is followed, no supplementary purified fibers are necessary.

You can double or treble your fiber intake by eating bran or wholegrain cereals (such as All-Bran®, oatmeal, porridge, shredded wheat and Grape-nuts®), wholegrain or wholemeal bread, more beans and vegetables.

Fiber and your blood sugar

After a high-fiber meal your blood sugar is not as high as after one low in fiber. One of the first people to write about this in the scientific journals was Dr David Jenkins of Oxford University in England who studied the blood sugar responses of diabetic patients after high and low-fiber meals. Before both types of meal, their blood sugars averaged 160 mg per 100 ml (9 mmol per liter); after low-fiber meals, the blood sugar quickly rose to 380 mg per 100 ml (21 mmol per liter) and remained above 300 mg per 100 ml (14 mmol per liter) for about two hours.

When high-fiber meals were taken, the blood sugar slowly went up to 260 mg per 100 ml (14 mmol per liter) and then returned slowly to the original level. This lowering of blood sugar is because fibers slow down and smooth out the absorption of sugars and starches from the intestine. In addition, less glucose is lost in the urine.

We can compare wholemeal or graham flour to highly refined cake flour: wholemeal flour is used to make a wholesome bread which retains its natural flavour and has a crunchy or nutty character; whereas cake flour and sugar are used to make a white bakery cake.

One small slice of graham or wholemeal bread has about 50 calories, many retained vitamins and minerals and is usually eaten slowly as part of a meal. One slice of cake has about 300 calories, and can be eaten very quickly without chewing. Once you've eaten a slice of cake, you'll probably still feel hungry. In a diabetic patient, after one slice of wholemeal bread, the blood sugar may rise by 10 or 20 mg per 100 ml ($\frac{1}{2}$ to 1 mmol per liter); after one slice of cake it may rise by 100 to 150 mg per 100 ml ($5\frac{1}{2}$ to 8 mmol per liter). So it's easy to see which is better for you to eat.

Fiber will lower your blood fats

Blood fats as mentioned in chapter five consist of cholesterol and triglycerides. Over many years raised blood fats can cause hardening of the arteries and eventually lead to heart attack or stroke.

For non-diabetics, insulin regulates the way in which fat is broken down by the body. With inadequate insulin too much cholesterol and triglycerides are retained by the body, and for this reason diabetics are especially vulnerable to high blood fat levels leading to hardening of the arteries.

Fibers with the jello-like (jelly) property that dissolves and absorbs water are able to lower your cholesterol levels. We have also found that a high-fiber diet is effective in lowering high blood fats and will also help you to lose weight as an added bonus. You should also avoid alcohol, at least until the diet has its full effect.

Traditional diets for diabetics

In many ways the high-fiber diet plans we have developed are the opposite of the traditional diabetic diets. Our high-fiber diets restrict fat and encourage starch carbohydrate intake, whereas the traditional programs required large amounts of fat and restricted carbohydrates of all types.

The reason for this was that over the centuries doctors developed the (incorrect) theory that the best diabetic diets were exceptionally low in carbohydrate but very high in fat and cholesterol. They thought that if your body had difficulty in burning off the energy from sugars due to insufficient insulin then you should cut out both table sugar and all other carbohydrates such as starches which are broken down into sugars. There were no scientific experiments to support this theory.

In 1925 many diabetic patients were treated with diets containing a staggering 200 g (7 oz) of fat, 1500 mg ($1\frac{1}{2}$ oz) of cholesterol and only 40 g of carbohydrate. In 1928 Dr Elliott P. Joslin, of the world-famous Boston Diabetes Clinic, warned that eating enormous quantities of fat and cholesterol may cause hardening of the arteries.

These very high-fat diets were also hard to follow, as people got tired of heavy cream, butter without bread, steak without potatoes, and eggs without toast. Besides, some diabetics ate fairly normal diets and seemed to do well. Gradually more and more carbohydrate was allowed. By 1955 many diabetic patients were eating almost 200 g (7 oz) of carbohydrate without difficulty. Consequently, by 1970 most diabetes experts recommended that diabetics could safely eat as much carbohydrate as non-diabetics. Table sugar, or sucrose, however, was still banned from the diet.

It now looks as though these traditional diets may have increased heart attacks and strokes among diabetic patients. Diabetic gangrene is a hundred times more common among American than Japanese diabetics. Heart attacks and strokes are about five times more common in American than in Japanese diabetics. As the Japanese diet has very little fat or cholesterol, this may protect Japanese diabetics from hardening of the arteries. The potential disadvantages of traditional western diabetic diets led us to consider a quite different approach to dieting. Our development of high-fiber diets is outlined in chapter eight.

Dietetic foods
There is a wide enough selection of foods without going to the dietetic section of your supermarket. In general, dietetic foods are expensive and, in my opinion, not worth the prices charged. Unsweetened canned fruits and bottled dressings can be useful. I advise my patients to avoid buying dietetic candies and desserts.

Fruits can be packed in water, artificially sweetened, packed in their own juice or packed in syrup (meaning added sugar); those packed in water or artificially sweetened have far fewer calories than those packed in juice or syrup and I recommend these. However, if you find an exceptional bargain in your favorite fruit packed in syrup, you can buy it and follow this procedure which eliminates most of the added sugar: pour off all the syrup and rinse the fruit thoroughly in cold water; let it stand for 30 minutes in cold water, rinse several times with water and refrigerate.

The label 'reduced calorie' on salad dressing indicates that instead of 45 calories per tablespoon of the regular dressing, it has less than 15 calories per tablespoon.

Artificial sweeteners
My patients often express their concern about saccharine, the only non-caloric sweetener currently available. (Cyclamates are still available in some other countries, outside the United States.) After weighing up the potential risks against the benefits, I tell my adult patients they can use saccharine in moderation, but I recommend them to limit intake to two servings a day (equal to two diet colas or four packets of artificial

sweetener or four sweetener pills). I advise pregnant women to avoid saccharin entirely and children to limit their intake to an occasional diet cola. I personally have switched from having a diet cola with my lunch to canned tomato juice which has only 42 calories per 180 g (6 oz) serving.

Products made from fructose or high fructose corn sweeteners are perfectly safe, but they are simple carbohydrates of the type we limit in our diabetic diets. My main concern about products containing fructose and corn syrup is their relatively high calorie content. For this reason I don't recommend candies, cookies, cakes or icings made from these sugars; fruit is much better. Three sugar alcohols (sorbitol, mannitol and xylitol) are used in certain products; in chewing gum they are less likely to lead to cavities than sucrose, but otherwise they have few other advantages.

Alcohol
Not many of my patients ask my advice about alcohol, but when they ask me I tell them that alcohol in moderation (less than 60 ml or 2 fluid oz per day) may not be hazardous for their health. But if you take insulin you should stick to the following precautions: Don't drink alcohol on an empty stomach as it lowers your blood sugar. Always eat something before drinking. Limit your alcohol intake to less than 60 ml (2 fluid oz) per day as excessive amounts may cause low blood sugars and lead to errors in your insulin dose or food intake.

7 ARE YOU OVERWEIGHT?

Obesity is now so common that in North America and most developed countries it is regarded as the number one health problem; the focus has clearly shifted from under-nutrition and deficiency to over-nutrition and diseases of excess. Being obese or very overweight not only reduces our life expectancy, it makes life far less enjoyable. If you are overweight you are subjected to jokes and may lose both your self-respect and self-confidence. You may lack energy, fall asleep easily and have a variety of minor complaints related to your weight. We all have a certain amount of gluttony within us that we must constantly fight to control. It has been estimated that about 75 per cent of all adults with diabetes are overweight. So if you are diabetic and overweight you will have much more difficulty controlling your blood sugar level.

Doctors define obesity as weighing 20 per cent more than your lean or desirable weight. You can of course be overweight anywhere between your lean weight and 20 per cent over. You can estimate your lean body weight as follows. First, measure your height in inches, in bare feet (most people shrink as they grow older; your present height is what matters). Second, if you are a woman allow 100 lb (45 kg) for 5 ft and 5 lb (2 kg) for each additional inch above 5 ft. So if you are 5 ft 4 in tall you should weigh about 120 lb (100 plus 20) (54 kg). If you are a man, allow 115 lb for 5 ft and again, add 5 lb for each inch above 5 ft. So if you are 5 ft 8 in tall you should weigh about 155 lb (115 plus 40) (69 kg).

These estimates do not make allowance for age, body frame and athletic training. Because of the wide variation in body type, some doctors now try to arrive at a lean weight by measuring the skin fold thicknesses in different parts of the body for even greater accuracy.

You can estimate how close you are to your lean weight as follows: Weigh yourself before breakfast, wearing very light clothing, divide your own weight by your estimated lean weight; multiply by 100 to get the percentage. For example, if you weigh 150 lb (68 kg) and your lean weight is 120 lb (54 kg) – 150 divided by 120 equals 1.25; 1.25 times 100 equals 125 per cent. You weigh 25 per cent above your lean or desirable weight. You are rather overweight!

A weight-loss strategy

Simply, to lose weight you must eat less food. Occasionally people can lose weight by doing more exercise. In my opinion there are four elements to a good weight reduction program, listed in my order of priority.
1. A motivated patient who wants to lose weight and who is also encouraged by his close family.
2. A supportive therapist (doctor, dietitian, or behavior therapist).
3. A weight-reducing diet.
4. A regular exercise program.

I have treated hundreds of overweight patients in the hospital, with great success. The problem with obesity is keeping the weight off. A thousand fad diets will help you lose weight, but you cannot follow a fad diet for ever. Being overweight is like being an alcoholic. You must stop overeating and stay off it for the rest of your life.

A motivated patient

Motivated patients are committed to losing weight and to keeping their weight down. Being committed is being dedicated in the strongest possible way. Most overweight patients have lost and regained weight a dozen times. We call this the yo-yo phenomenon, and it is more harmful to your health than maintaining the same overweight state.

From my experience you have three options. First, you can make a strong commitment to lose weight and become involved in a sensible program that will help you lose weight, and keep it off. There are many good programs, some directed by physicians or health professionals, while others are businesses (Weight Watchers for instance). Second, you can enjoy life and not worry about your weight. Third, you can jump from one fad diet to another. You can always lose weight with some fad diet, as most rely on large losses of water during the first two weeks. Losses of water, however, are temporary, and as soon as you deviate from the fad diet you will regain the water your body needs. Obviously, I think the first option is the best for your health, but anyway the second option is better than the third. The encouragement of your close family is vital for you to lose weight. Often being overweight is a family problem; it's difficult to diet if the rest of the family are a crowd of gluttons!

A supportive therapist

Most people can lose weight more readily if they relate to a good therapist. Your therapist can be a doctor, dietitian, another health professional or a team which specializes in weight reduction. Your therapist should sincerely believe that you can lose weight and work with you in a sympathetic and supportive way. You'll need to see him or her at regular intervals. Behavior modification techniques to help you eat less food are used successfully by some groups, and are of great help to some people.

A weight-reducing diet

Obesity, diabetes and alcoholism are lifelong problems for which there are no miracle cures. There are no magic diets for losing weight, and some fad diets (such as protein-modified fasting) are actually dangerous. I get my patients to use a well-balanced, health-maintaining diet. Initially, calories are moderately restricted to ensure a good rate of weight loss. As my patients approach their desired weight, the caloric content of the diet is increased. When they reach a lean weight the calories are increased to maintain it. We use high-fiber, generous carbohydrate diets. Initially our patients receive intensive instruction in the use of these diets; at every check-up they receive further information and reinforcement.

A regular exercise program

To lose weight your body must burn more calories than you eat. To do this, you can eat less food, or you can burn more calories through exercise and physical activity. To lose weight adequately you must do both. If you can burn 450 extra calories a day you'll manage to lose an extra pound in weight a week – walking after meals is excellent for this. You use about one-third of your calories every day in digesting and absorbing your food. Exercise during this digestive process uses up extra calories. For example, walking *before* you eat may burn 100 calories, whereas walking the same distance *after* meals may use 150 calories. Exercise also contributes to your health by lowering your blood sugar and blood fats, strengthening your muscles and giving you more vigor and vitality.

If you take insulin or pills

As weight loss lowers your blood sugar, you may not need as much insulin or as many pills to treat your diabetes. In my experience most overweight patients on insulin can adequately control their diabetes with much lower doses or even no insulin at all if they lose weight and follow a diet; and those on antidiabetic pills usually can stop them altogether. Often my patients can reduce their insulin dose by 10 per cent each week if all urine tests (measured four times daily) are free of sugar.

High-fiber weight-reducing diets

Some of our patients have lost weight nicely on high-fiber diets. We have been able to stop their insulin, and their blood sugars and fats are much lower.

These diets have several features which help weight reduction. They have restricted amounts of fat and sugar, both of which are big sources of calories but aren't very filling. The high-fiber content provides satiety, a feeling of fullness and satisfaction. The caloric density of the foods is low; but because of their bulky content you need to eat more of the food to get the same number of calories. Some of these high-fiber foods have to be chewed more, so the meals take longer to eat. These diets have all been carefully analyzed in our laboratories. Over the last few years we have been able to accumulate plenty of practical experience in using these diets to help patients to lose weight. Even with this experience, we know that to lose weight you'll not only need to follow the diets closely but also keep off the foods not recommended.

In the hospital, we have used 800 calorie high-fiber diets, which allow us to reduce insulin doses rapidly in most cases. Many patients lose 5 to 8 lb (2.25–3.50 kg) during the first week in hospital. Overweight patients who are taking over 50 units of insulin per day are usually hospitalized to begin the diet. For home use, we usually use 1000, 1200 or 1500 calorie diets, a 1000 calorie diet for a woman weighing about 150 lb (68 kg) who should weigh 110 lb (50 kg), and a 1500 calorie diet for a man weighing over 250 lb (113 kg). Sample diets are supplied in the *Guide to HCF diets* which begins on page 109.

8 ARE HIGH-FIBER DIETS FOR YOU?

Around 1970 we became interested in high-fiber diets because of the limitations of traditional diabetic diets. Over the last ten years we developed the high-carbohydrate, high-fiber (which we abbreviate to HCF) diets; we have been using them for over six years now and find them to be safe and well-tolerated by our patients.

Since our team's findings were published in the *American Journal of Clinical Nutrition* in 1976, we have been inundated with several thousand requests for detailed information from all over the world. In response to this, I am setting out here the key features of this diet which was developed at a major teaching hospital, with all patients closely supervised by my staff and myself.

Before starting the HCF diet, it is important that you consult your doctor. The diet has been modified for home use – for example, the amount of daily fiber recommended in the home HCF diet is two-thirds of that contained in the hospital diet. Also, while our patients are in the hospital, we only give them 30 g (1 oz) of meat each day compared to about 150 g (5 oz) when they get home. Our patients find this modified diet plan more convenient and practical for their day-to-day living. Most of my patients have found that the HCF diet has worked so well for them in hospital – both for control of their diabetes and for the way they feel in general – that they are motivated to continue it when they get home.

Why HCF diets are good for anyone

These diets lower insulin needs and blood fat levels; you will benefit further if you cut down your intake of animal fat and cholesterol. Most adults, both diabetic and non-diabetic, would be healthier on these diets.

HCF diets for adult-type diabetics
Every patient that we have treated with the HCF diet has gained some improvement in his or her diabetes, and those with the adult-type have had the best results. We have been able to discontinue insulin therapy in 18 out of 20 patients taking less than 25 units of insulin per day, and they have

been able to remain off insulin for up to four years if they follow the diet very closely. In 15 patients who were receiving between 25 and 40 units of insulin per day, we have been able to stop insulin therapy in slightly more than half (8 out of 15).

The two groups of patients described above were not overweight; these reductions in insulin doses occurred without weight loss. The diets work much better for overweight patients who lose weight on them. I feel that a prudent diabetic diet should contain 55 to 60 per cent of calories from carbohydrate, about 15 per cent from protein and less than 30 per cent as fat. A 1500 calorie diet provides per day about 240 g (8 oz) carbohydrate, 60 g (2 oz) of protein, 44 g ($1\frac{1}{2}$ oz) of fat, less than 150 mg ($\frac{1}{200}$ oz) of cholesterol and 50 g ($1\frac{1}{2}$ oz) of plant fiber. A sample 1500 calorie menu plan is given in the *Guide to HCF diets*, which begins on page 109.

HCF diets for juvenile-type diabetics
We have treated less than a dozen patients with this type of diabetes with HCF diets. The diets lower insulin needs by an average of 25 per cent. These patients, by definition, are totally dependent on insulin and cannot stop their insulin injections with any type of diet. In half of the patients, we feel that diabetic control is distinctly better; they have on average fewer insulin reactions and better blood sugars. Also blood cholesterol levels drop in every patient and this may be a major plus. My colleagues from other medical centers have successfully used these diets to treat children with juvenile-type diabetes. However, I have not yet treated children with HCF diets so I can't tell you about their usefulness for diabetics under twenty years old.

Practical hints for HCF diets

Family
Many of my patients ask whether the diet is good for their whole family. I tell them that it is a wholesome diet for anyone, so there's no need to prepare two meals – one for you and one for the rest of your family. You won't feel isolated on your special diet. After a couple of weeks, your family will also enjoy it. Growing children, up to fourteen years old for girls and sixteen for boys, should be given larger servings of meat, up to 180 to 240 g (6 or 8 oz) and several glasses of milk each day.

Shopping
Most of the foods on the diet can be bought at supermarkets, and you will probably save between 20 and 30 per cent on your weekly grocery bill, as you'll be buying less meat, convenience foods and candy.

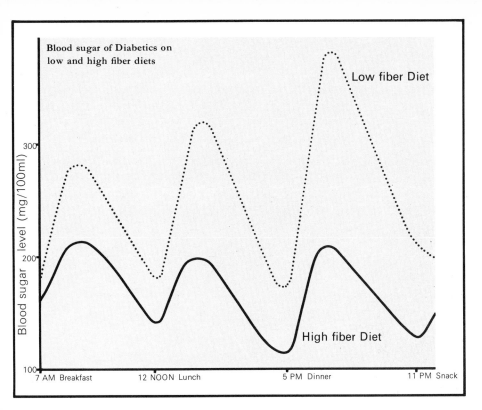

Blood sugar of Diabetics on low and high fiber diets

Low fiber Diet

High fiber Diet

Blood sugar level (mg/100ml)

300

200

100

7 AM Breakfast   12 NOON Lunch   5 PM Dinner   11 PM Snack

When buying bread always look carefully to check the type of flour used. High-fiber breads are made with wholewheat or wholemeal (graham) flour; if you buy from a bakery, check to see that more wholewheat than refined, white flour has been used. Wholewheat spaghetti and noodles are also now becoming more widely available.

Steer clear of foods with added sugar and excess fat. Most people know that foods like butter, lard, margarine, and vegetable oils contain visible fats. Far fewer are aware of the large amount of invisible fat they eat in food such as cheeses, lean meats (about 20 to 30 per cent fat), mayonnaise, salad dressings, potato chips and crisps, peanut butter, nuts, olives, chocolate, cakes and pastries. White fish and poultry contain far less fat than red meat. If you like cheese, several low-fat cheeses are available in North America such as uncreamed cottage cheese, farmer's cheese (low fat curd cheese), and part-skimmed mozarella cheese.

Fruit and vegetables are also an important part of our diet. Try to use those that are available and in season. If fresh fruits are not in season, use those frozen without added sugar or canned without sugar, the water-packed variety. Avoid vegetables which are canned or frozen with sauces and other fatty ingredients. Quite often you can find vegetables that are frozen without any additives at all.

Common problems with HCF diets

These diets do produce gas. Everyone knows that eating beans causes gas. Recently medical research has discovered that it is the fiber in beans that causes this. When the fiber reaches the large intestine known as the colon, it is fermented or burned by bacteria, which produces flatulence (passing gas below) or belching. There is, however, no bloating or discomfort, and patients adjust to increased amounts of gas and find ways to expel it that are not embarrassing.

For the first few days on HCF diets you may notice some abdominal fullness and some difficulty eating all the food planned for you, but this will disappear after you adjust to a much larger intake of bulk. None of our patients have had to stop HCF diets because of discomfort or side-effects. With these diets you will be exchanging a lot of problems, such as high blood sugars, unhealthy blood fat levels, or constipation, for minor nuisances such as belching and flatulence.

Other special HCF diets

HCF diets for blood cholesterol problems

If your blood cholesterol exceeds 300 mg per 100 ml (17 mmol per liter), your chances of a heart attack are about three times higher than someone your age and sex with a cholesterol count below 180 mg per 100 ml.

Emil, a forty-seven year-old book-keeper was in the high-risk category. His father and two brothers had heart attacks before the age of fifty and all of them had cholesterol problems. Emil's cholesterol had been between 300 and 350 mg per 100 ml (17 and 19 mmol per liter) for the past five years. Last year he started having chest pain related to a blockage around his heart. He was hospitalized for treatment with our HCF diet. In two weeks his blood cholesterol dropped from 306 mg per 100 ml to 170 mg per 100 ml (17 to 9 mmol per liter), the lowest value ever recorded in his family. He went home on a liberalized diet which contained oat bran and dried beans; six weeks later his cholesterol was 163 mg per 100 ml (9 mmol per liter), a new record low value for his family. Over the next six months he followed the diet closely and all cholesterol readings were below 180 mg per 100 ml (10 mmol per liter). Statistically, the diet has greatly lowered his risk for a heart attack.

HCF diets for blood triglyceride problems

Triglycerides (storage forms of fat) accumulate in the blood of some people and contribute to hardening of the arteries. The following case history shows how triglyceride problems can be controlled.

Richard, a fifty-three year-old automobile mechanic, was sent to see me because his blood triglyceride values were above 3000 mg per 100 ml (162 mmol per liter) (over 20 times the normal). He was overweight but did not drink alcohol. We hospitalized him immediately to control these dangerously high blood triglycerides. With the HCF diet his triglycerides dropped over 2000 points in a week. Over the next four months he lost 35 lb (15 kg) and his triglyceride values fell to less than 300 mg per 100 ml (17 mmol per liter). He has maintained a reasonable weight on a high-fiber diet and over the past two years his triglycerides have averaged 300 mg per 100 ml (17 mmol per liter).

The high-fiber diet we use to treat triglyceride problems is identical to that we use for diabetic patients. Getting down to a trim body weight using diet and exercise usually controls the problems. Alcohol should be avoided.

Non-diabetic hypoglycemia

The blood sugar of non-diabetics often drops after a meal, especially one low in fiber. The pre-meal level of blood sugar starts at about 80 mg per 100 ml (4 mmol per liter). After a typical low-fiber meal, the blood sugar rises 30 to 50 points to a peak of about 120 mg per 100 ml (7 mmol per liter). Then it falls to its lowest level of between 60 and 70 mg per 100 ml (3 and 4 mmol per liter). So, you can see that for a short time the blood sugar drops 10 or 20 mg per 100 ml ($\frac{1}{2}$ to 1 mmol per liter) below the pre-meal level. This commonly happens to normal non-diabetics with no problems, although if they have abnormalities in their stomach emptying this can also cause hypoglycemia.

If, for instance, the stomach rapidly dumps food into the small intestine, excessive insulin may be released from the pancreas, which can cause the blood sugar to drop rapidly to abnormally low values. Stomach-emptying problems can occur after stomach surgery, but also in people who have never had surgery. In both situations, the blood sugar reaches its lowest values between one-and-a-half and three hours after the meal.

Hypoglycemia is now becoming a popular topic for discussion. *Time* magazine recently called it a fad disease because most people have some of the problems or symptoms listed above. Only occasionally patients have the hypoglycemia which is at the root of their symptoms. Nevertheless, it is a real problem for some people and I have treated many non-diabetic patients who had genuine hypoglycemia. However, I use very strict criteria to establish that hypoglycemia is a problem in a patient. I need to be able to see all three of the following:

1. Troublesome symptoms between meals.
2. A documented plasma glucose value below 45 mg per 100 ml ($2\frac{1}{2}$ mmol per liter) after a meal or glucose test.
3. A recurrence of the troublesome symptoms when the blood sugar is low.

When I see all three of these features, I tell my patients that they have hypoglycemia which can be overcome by vigorous dietary management. Our western diets, with large amounts of sugar and very little fiber, foster the development of hypoglycemia; it is very rare in countries where sugar consumption is low and fiber intake is high.

If you have non-diabetic hypoglycemia, you should completely avoid sucrose and simple sugars such as fruit juices, cola drinks, candies, cookies, cakes and honey. You should limit your milk intake (the sugar in milk is lactose) to half a cup a day and only eat one or two pieces of fruit a day until your condition is greatly improved. We limit the intake of simple carbohydrates (sucrose and simple sugars) to 50 g ($1\frac{1}{2}$ oz) per day, most of it from vegetables, small servings of milk and limited amounts of fresh fruits. We encourage a generous intake of fiber from bran and wholegrain cereals such as oatmeal (porridge), All-Bran®, Grapenuts®, and shredded wheat; wholegrain breads and crackers such as rye crisps or crispbread; beans, such as pinto beans; garden vegetables such as carrots, corn, green beans, peas and tomatoes; and starchy vegetables like potatoes and rice.

The best diet for treating hypoglycemia bears a surprising resemblance to that for treating diabetes. Both are HCF, limited in sucrose and simple sugars. (We have carefully tested high-protein diets and do not find them beneficial for our patients.) Most diets consist of three meals per day plus a bedtime snack; after a stomach operation six small meals per day are advisable. This HCF diet works well for all types of hypoglycemia that follows meals. In my experience drugs and injections are better avoided in treating hypoglycemia. Over the past five years all my patients have responded well to these diets without use of any drug therapy. Diets which we have used successfully for our patients are given in the next chapter.

If you have hypoglycemia, there is a high probability that a high-fiber, restricted sugar diet will correct your problems. But you must follow the diet meticulously for at least six weeks to see any improvement. Within two weeks you should feel better, but it may take a full three months on the diet to completely eliminate any symptoms of hypoglycemia. A sugar-eating 'binge' may set your progress back for several weeks. The investment of your time and effort, however, will pay dividends.

9 FOOD EXCHANGES

I think the diabetic's motto should be: 'Variety is the spice of life'. Diabetic patients often eat a greater variety of food than their non-diabetic friends, as the diabetes education process introduces them to many different foods. They can select a varied menu and still maintain a well-balanced diet. The non-diabetic, without the benefit of this nutrition education, may eat a rather routine diet which lacks variety. The key to these interesting food choices is *food exchanges*. Exchanging is a fancy word for trading or bartering – you can trade one fruit for another fruit, or one type of cereal for another type. In Australia they call diabetic exchanges 'substitutes'.

In our program, foods are divided into ten different food groups or exchanges: milk, A vegetables (low calorie), B vegetables, C vegetables (starchy), beans, breakfast cereals, bread, fruit, meat and fat. They have been planned so one serving of a food in the exchange lists at the end of the chapter, properly measured out, will give approximately the same number of calories and amount of carbohydrate, protein and fat as any other serving on the same list. Below are some exchanges for breakfast foods. From this you can see how simple and varied the exchanges are. However, I strongly advise you to consult your own doctor before you change your existing exchange diet.

Your meal plan may allow these for breakfast:
>1 cereal exchange
>1 milk exchange
>1 fruit exchange
>2 bread exchanges
>1 fat exchange

For breakfast on Monday you could have:
>oatmeal (porridge)
>skim milk
>orange juice
>wholewheat toast
>margarine

For breakfast on Tuesday you could have:
    shredded wheat
    skim milk
    grapefruit
    corn muffin
    margarine

For breakfast on Wednesday you could have:
    yogurt with fruit
    graham crackers or crispbread

For breakfast on Thursday you could have:
    Grapenuts® or Bran Buds®
    skim milk
    banana
    wholewheat toast
    margarine

These are simple examples. On other days, you could have waffles, pancakes or French toast. If you like eggs and sausage for breakfast our diet would allow scrambled egg whites or scrambled egg substitutes (such as Egg Beaters® in North America) plus a breakfast pattie (such as Morning Star Farm® in North America). A sample meal plan for a full day is given in the *Guide to HCF diets*, which starts on page 109.

All the foods in one group are similar and each group gives you all the daily requirements for good nutrition. All the fruits in the fruit exchange have about the same number of calories; foods in the cereal exchange have similar amounts of carbohydrate, protein and fat, and those in the vegetable exchange have equal amounts of fiber. Thus each food exchange contains a number of food equivalents. Because most exchanges have dozens of different foods, you can have an enormous variety, and your meals will not be monotonous. A list of ten food exchanges are given in the *Guide to food exchanges* section later in this chapter.

A tailormade food plan

Your doctor or dietitian will help you develop a diet that meets your energy needs and other special requirements. This plan will be tailored to your likes and dislikes as far as possible; if, for example, you don't like cucumber, you can delete it from your food exchange list.

1. The first thing to decide is how many calories you need. If you are lean, you can estimate your caloric needs as follows. If you are not active (you sit at a desk all day), multiply your body weight in pounds by 12; this gives you an approximation of your daily caloric needs. For example, if you weigh 120 lb (54 kg), $120 \times 12 = 1440$, or 1440 calories. This only applies if you are lean or skinny.

   Younger people will require more calories and older people far fewer.

   If you are moderately active (you work in a factory for instance), multiply your body weight by 15; if you weigh 140 lb (63 kg) for example, $140 \times 15 = 2100$ calories.

   If you are very active (a farmer or furniture-mover, for example), multiply your weight by 18. If for example, you weigh 150 lb (67 kg), $150 \times 18 = 2700$ calories. In my experience most middle-aged women need between 10 to 13 calories per lb and most middle-aged men need 11 to 15 calories per lb. (This 11–15 calories per lb is equivalent to 100 to 140 kJ per kg.)

2. The second decision is how much carbohydrate and protein you need. Usually we give about 55 per cent carbohydrate and 18 per cent protein of total calories; fat fills in the remaining calories (27 per cent in this example). A 1500 calorie diet would give you 206 g (7 oz) of carbohydrate, 68 g (2 oz) of protein and 45 g ($1\frac{1}{2}$ oz) of fat, calculated as follows: For carbohydrate 1500 calories $\times$ 55 per cent = 825 calories; carbohydrate has 4 calories per gram – 825 calories divided by 4 = 206 g (7 oz). For protein 1500 calories $\times$ 18 per cent = 270 calories; protein has 4 calories per gram – 270 divided by 4 = 68 g (2 oz). For fat 1500×27 per cent = 405 calories; fat has 9 calories per gram – 405 divided by 9 = 45 g ($1\frac{1}{2}$ oz). Our exchange plan provides a good fiber intake and a low cholesterol level.

3. To develop your food plan, the grams of carbohydrate, protein and fat must be converted into exchanges, and your food preferences and eating habits taken into account. I will explain how this is done later in this chapter.

4. These food exchanges are now assigned to different meals and snacks. Your doctor or dietitian will tell you how many servings from each group to have at each meal. If you take insulin, you may need snacks at special times. I have given meal plan examples for different calorie levels in the *Guide to HCF diets* in this chapter, com-

mencing on page 109. I hope these will give you and your family an idea of how appetizing and varied they are. Always remember though that following the meal plans isn't enough. You are unique and have special needs and there's no way that a book can take account of this. Your doctor or dietitian must supervise your diet and the way you control your diabetes. Once your personal diet has been developed, you should follow it carefully.

How to calculate your exchanges
To figure out the number of servings for each exchange, you and your dietitian should take a sheet of paper and make a table like the one below with the names of the ten exchanges on the left hand side. Make column headings across the top for servings, carbohydrate, protein, fat and fiber. At the bottom of the table enter the gram values for carbohydrate, protein and fat (the *target values*) you calculated in under 2 above (don't worry about the fiber until you have finished the other calculations). You will need at least one milk serving, three to five meat servings, one to three servings of each type of vegetable (A, B, and C) at least one serving each of cereal and beans, and between three and eight servings of bread, fruit and fat.

Use a pencil with a good eraser when you work out your plan. Enter the number of servings that you would like from each exchange per day. Then write down how many grams of carbohydrate, protein and fat these foods would give you. (These values for each exchange are given in the *Guide to food exchanges* later on in this chapter.) Add up the totals to see how closely you match the target figures already entered at the bottom line.

The actual total should be very close (within 1 to 3 g) to your target. You'll need to keep changing the exchanges until the actual total matches the target values. After you have finished this process you can enter the values for fiber and add up how much fiber will be in your diet.

Which foods can you eat?

I want to summarize here the different types of exchanges in the meal plan. In the *Guide to food exchanges* section further on, you'll find a wide selection of foods set out under the heading of each of the following types of exchanges.

Milk exchanges
Milk is one of the important basic foods which you should have every day. It is an important source of protein, calcium and several vitamins. You

Exchanges	Servings	Carbohydrate	Protein	Fat	Fiber
Milk	1	11	8	0.5	0
A vegetable	2	4	2	0	4
B vegetable	2	8	4	0	4
C vegetable	2	30	4	1	6
Beans	1	12	7	0.5	8
Cereal	1	13	2	0.5	3
Bread	6	66	12	6	10
Fruit	6	60	0	0	12
Meat	4	0	32	8	0
Fat	6	0	0	27	0
Actual total, as grams		204	71	44	47
Target, as grams		*206*	*68*	*45*	—

should only use skim milk, skim milk powder or evaporated skim milk. Other milk products such as yogurt should not contain more than 1 g of fat per exchange.

Vegetables
Using a wide variety of vegetables promotes good health and vitality. While most vegetables are low in calories, they provide fiber and a variety of vitamins and minerals. Also the variety of colors and flavors of vegetables will help to make your diet interesting as well as satisfying.

Vegetables may be bought in any form – either fresh, frozen or canned, but should not have fat, sauces, cheeses, glazes, sugar or similar seasonings added. Preparation of vegetable casseroles will help you use a variety of different vegetables and may replace meat dishes that contain more fat.

Bean exchanges
Beans provide an excellent source of protein, carbohydrate, minerals and fiber. The fiber in beans is also particularly useful in lowering the blood cholesterol concentration. Using beans as a source of protein cuts out the saturated fats and cholesterol we get from meat. Some of your meat allowances such as ham can be used to season beans and improve the quality of protein that you eat. Combining beans with rice or other grains also improves the quality of protein that you are getting.

Cereal exchanges

Cereals are an excellent source of fiber and also provide vitamins and minerals. Some of the high fiber breakfast cereals on the market contain too much sugar. We have chosen cereals which provide an adequate amount of fiber and do not, in our opinion, have too much sugar. You may want to use some of your fruit or fruit juice allowance instead of an artificial sweetener to sweeten your cereal. Cereals need not be limited to breakfast but also make good bedtime snacks.

Bread exchanges

You should shop for breads, crackers and crispbread that have whole-grain or graham flour such as stoneground or wholewheat flour as the main ingredient. The labels on breads should be checked carefully to see if wholegrain or wholewheat flour is the first and therefore main ingredient. While it is rarely possible to find commercial breads not containing sugar, honey or molasses, these should not be principal ingredients. Whenever you can, choose bread baked with vegetable fat, rather than butter.

Fruit exchanges

Fruits are natural desserts. They satisfy your sweet tooth but do not add refined sugar to your diet. They can be used in salads, for snacks and in your lunch box. Fruits are valuable sources of vitamins, minerals and fiber.

Choose fruits that are raw, canned in their own juice, unsweetened or artificially sweetened. Fruits are preferred to fruit juices as a fruit exchange because they contain more fiber. It is important to consider the size indicated for each exchange as some fruits contain more calories than others of comparable size.

Meat, fish and cheese exchanges

These are good sources of high quality protein. Very small servings of meat will complement the vegetable proteins and provide you with a well-balanced intake of important amino acids. Proteins from animal sources often provide excessive amounts of fat and cholesterol so you should limit your intake of meats and cheeses to reduce your dietary fat and cholesterol.

Your daily intake of meat, milk products, vegetables and cereal products will provide you with all the fat your body needs. We suggest to our patients that they limit their fat intake and use these fat exchanges for seasoning purposes and as dressings for salads. For variety we have included several kinds of nuts.

Guide to HCF diets

People sometimes think high-fiber meals are monotonous. I hope this section will show how varied and wholesome the HCF diet can be.

1800 CALORIE HCF MEAL PLAN

Meal	Exchanges	Food	Portion USA	UK
BREAKFAST	1 Milk	Skim milk	1 cup	7 oz
	1 Fruit	Orange	1 medium	1 oz
	1 Cereal	All Bran®	½ cup	2 tbs
	2 Bread	Wholewheat toast	2 slices	1½ oz
	2 Fat	Margarine	2 tsb	2 tsb
NOON MEAL	1 Meat	Pork	1 oz	1 oz
	2 Bread	Rye bread	2 slices	1½ oz
	1 Fat	Mayonnaise	1 tsp	1 tsp
	1 C Vegetable	Potatoes	½ cup	1 small
	1 Bean	Butter beans	½ cup	3 oz
	1 A Vegetable	Carrots	½ cup	3 oz
	1 Fruit	Canned peaches (water packed)	½ cup	2 halves
EVENING MEAL	1 Meat	Chicken	1 oz	1 oz
	2 Bread	Bran muffin	1	1
	1 A Vegetable	Green beans	½ cup	3 oz
	1 B Vegetable	Tomato	1 small	4 oz
	3 (USA) or 5 (UK) C Vegetable	Brown rice	1 cup	5 oz
	1 Bean	Haricot beans	½ cup	3 oz
	2 A Vegetables	Salad – cress, cucumber, lettuce		
SNACK	1 Fruit	Apple	½ large	1 medium
	2 Bread	Bran muffin	1	1

The quantities given in the two right-hand columns above are not exactly equivalent because American and British exchanges are calculated slightly differently. But both systems described here will give a well-balanced diet with around 1800 calories per day.

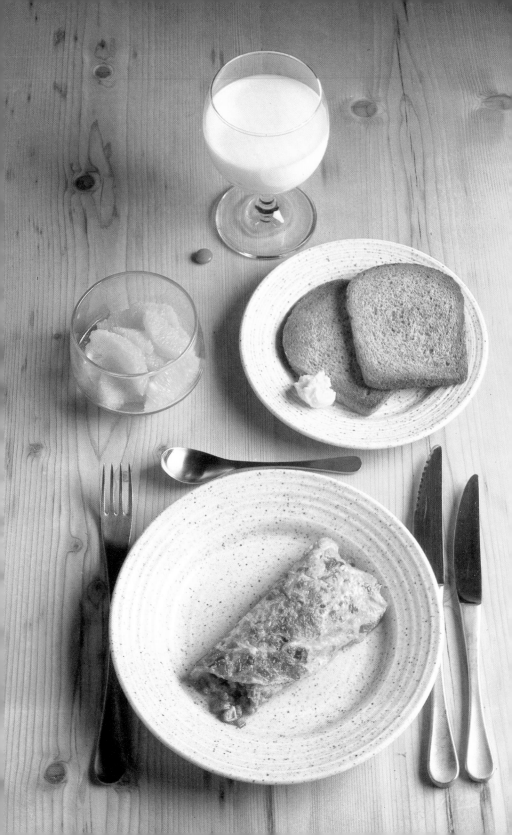

1500 CALORIE HIGH-FIBER MAINTENANCE DIET

This diet would be suitable for many women under 50 years old who weigh about 120–130 lb (54–59 kg) and also for overweight men who are trying to lose weight.

SUNDAY

BREAKFAST (*opposite*)	Spanish omelet Egg whites – 3 large Chopped green onion, green chili, pimento, green pepper Tomato paste or puree Orange slices – 1 orange Skim milk – 1 cup Whole wheat toast – 2 slices	Margarine – 1 tsp Multivitamin – 1
NOON MEAL	Dinner salad Lettuce – 1 cup Tomato – $\frac{1}{2}$ Cucumbers, radishes, celery, green onions, low calorie dressing Baked fish – 6 oz Brussels sprouts – $\frac{1}{2}$ cup Baked potato – 1 Roll, whole wheat – 1	Margarine – 1 tsp Fruit cocktail – $\frac{1}{2}$ cup
EVENING MEAL	Cole slaw Cabbage – $\frac{1}{2}$ cup Dressing – low fat Chili Chili powder Macaroni – $\frac{1}{2}$ cup Kidney beans – $\frac{1}{2}$ cup Tomatoes – $\frac{1}{2}$ cup Tomato juice – $\frac{1}{2}$ cup Chopped onion and	green pepper Rye crackers – 3 Margarine – 1 tsp Peaches, canned – $\frac{1}{2}$ cup
SNACK	Corn flakes – $\frac{3}{4}$ cup Skim milk – $\frac{1}{2}$ cup Banana – $\frac{1}{2}$ medium	

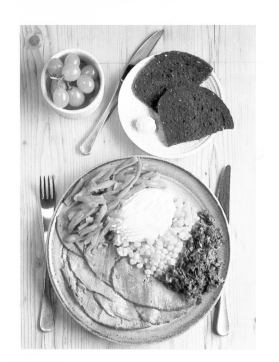

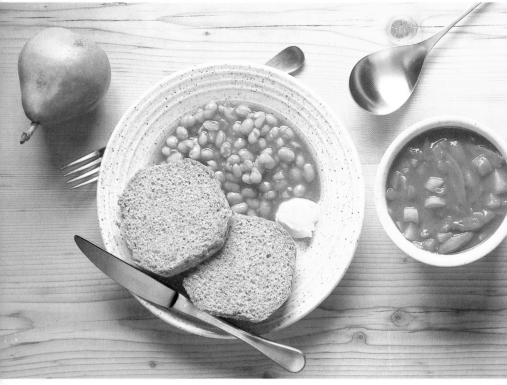

MONDAY

BREAKFAST	Oatmeal $-\frac{3}{4}$ cup (cooked) Skim milk $-$ 1 cup Orange juice $-\frac{1}{3}$ cup Whole wheat toast $-$ 1 slice Margarine $-$ 2 tsp Multivitamin $-$ 1

NOON MEAL
(*opposite below*)
	Vegetable soup
	  Tomato juice $-$ 1 cup
	  Potato, diced $-\frac{1}{2}$ cup
	  Onion, carrots, green
	  beans $-\frac{1}{2}$ cup
	  Bay leaf $-\frac{1}{2}$
	Baked beans $-\frac{1}{2}$ cup
	Bran muffin $-$ 1 (see recipe
	page 140)
	Margarine $-$ 1 tsp
	Pear $-$ 1

EVENING MEAL (*opposite above*)	Roast beef $-$ 4 oz Mashed potatoes $-\frac{1}{2}$ cup Corn $-\frac{1}{2}$ cup Green beans $-\frac{1}{2}$ cup Spinach $-\frac{1}{2}$ cup Rye bread $-$ 1 slice Margarine $-$ 1 tsp Grapes $-$ 10
SNACK	Carrot sticks Grapenuts® $-$ 3 tbs Strawberries $-$ 1 cup Skim milk $-\frac{1}{2}$ cup

TUESDAY

BREAKFAST

All Bran® – $\frac{1}{3}$ cup
  with banana – $\frac{1}{2}$
Skim milk – 1 cup
Apple juice – $\frac{1}{3}$ cup
Rye toast – 1 slice
Margarine – 1 tsp
Multivitamin – 1

NOON MEAL
(*opposite below*)

Turkey sandwich
  Turkey – 1 oz
  Rye bread – 2 slices
  Mayonnaise – 1 tsp
  Lettuce
Carrot sticks – $\frac{1}{2}$ cup
Tomato – 1 small
Green onions – 2
Cherries – 10 large

EVENING MEAL
(*opposite above*)

Dinner salad (see Sunday)
Broiled fish – 4 oz
Brown rice – $\frac{2}{3}$ cup
Navy beans – $\frac{1}{2}$ cup
Broccoli – $\frac{1}{2}$ cup
Beets – $\frac{1}{2}$ cup
Rye bread – 1 slice
Margarine – 1 tsp
Pears, canned – $\frac{1}{2}$ cup

SNACK

Shredded Wheat® – 1
biscuit
Skim milk – 1 cup
Rye bread – 1 slice
Margarine – 1 tsp

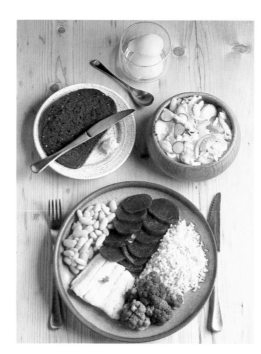

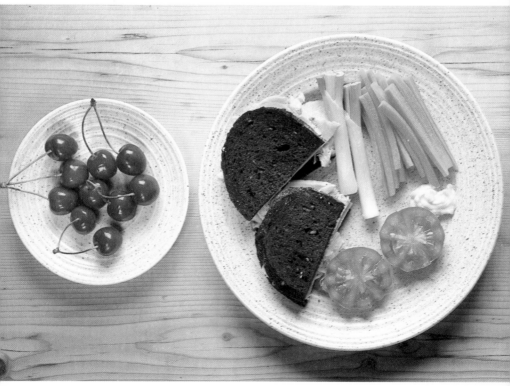

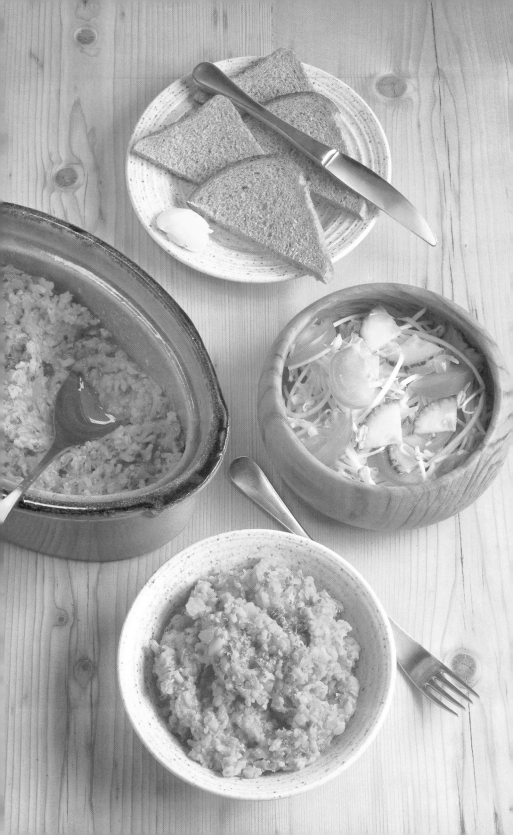

WEDNESDAY

BREAKFAST
Oatmeal – ¾ cup
   with raisins – 1½ tbs
Skim milk – ½ cup
Bran muffin – 1 (see recipe
page 140)
Margarine – 2 tsp
Pineapple juice – ⅓ cup

Multivitamin – 1

NOON MEAL
(*opposite*)
Sprout salad
   Bean sprouts – ½ cup
   Lettuce, cucumbers,
   tomatoes – ½ cup
   Low fat dressing
Savory lentil rice casserole*
   Lentils, cooked – ½ cup
   Brown rice, cooked – ⅔
   cup
   Tomato juice – ½ cup
   Onion, chopped – 1 tbs
   Beef bouillon
   Sweet basil – pinch
   (optional)

Whole wheat bread – 2
slices
Margarine – 1 tsp

EVENING MEAL
'Antipasta'
   Sticks of carrots, green
   pepper, celery stalks,
   sliced cucumbers, green
   onions, cauliflower,
   cherry tomatoes, olives
Roast turkey – 3 oz
Sweet potatoes, baked – ½
medium

Asparagus – ½ cup
Roll, whole wheat – 1
Margarine – 1 tsp

SNACK
Corn flakes – ¾ cup
Skim milk – ½ cup
Raspberries, canned – ½ cup

---

*Follow package directions for cooking lentils and brown rice. Mix cooked lentils, cooked brown rice, and onion well. Add basil to suit your taste. Add beef bouillon and tomato juice, mix well. Put into casserole dish. Cover and bake at 325°F for 30 minutes.

THURSDAY

BREAKFAST
(*opposite*)

Grapenut flakes® $-\frac{2}{3}$ cup
Skim milk $-\frac{1}{2}$ cup
Orange juice $-\frac{1}{3}$ cup
Whole wheat toast – 1 slice
Margarine – 1 tsp
Multivitamin – 1

NOON MEAL

Grapenut-fruit delight
   Grapenuts® – 3 tbs
   Yogurt, 2% fat – 5 oz
   Peaches, canned $-\frac{1}{4}$ cup
   Strawberries, frozen $-\frac{1}{2}$ cup
Graham crackers – 4 squares
Carrot sticks $-\frac{1}{2}$ cup
Green pepper sticks $-\frac{1}{2}$ cup

EVENING MEAL

Dinner salad (see Sunday)
Roast pork – 3 oz
Potatoes $-\frac{1}{2}$ cup
Margarine – 1 tsp
Corn on cob – 1 medium
Brussels sprouts $-\frac{1}{2}$ cup
Whole wheat bread – 1 slice
Margarine – 1 tsp
Apricots, canned $-\frac{1}{4}$ cup

SNACK

Plums – 2 small
Wheaties® $-\frac{1}{2}$ cup
Skim milk $-\frac{1}{2}$ cup
Carrot sticks $-\frac{1}{2}$ cup

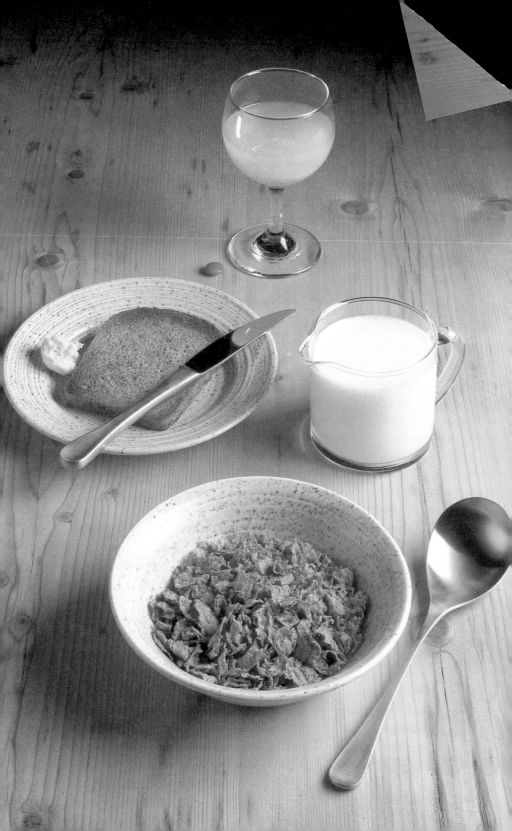

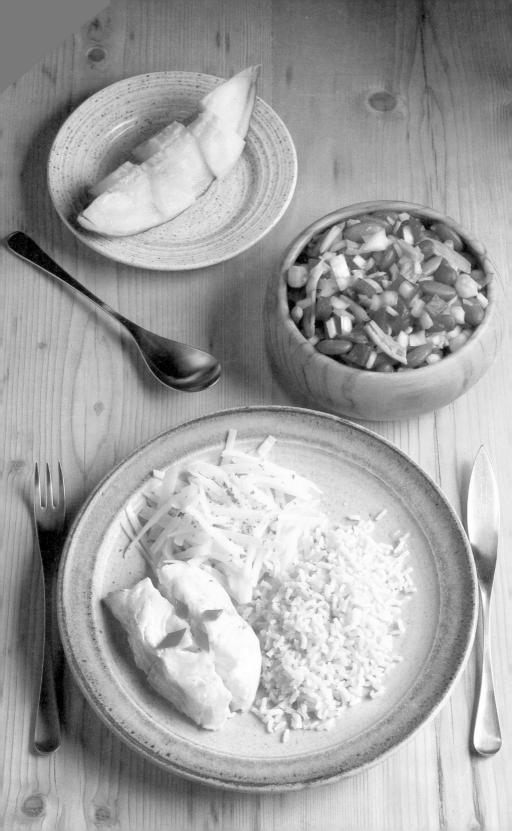

FRIDAY

BREAKFAST

Oatmeal $-\frac{1}{2}$ cup
  with Grapenuts® $-$ 1$\frac{1}{2}$ tbs
Skim milk $-\frac{1}{2}$ cup
Pineapple juice $-\frac{1}{3}$ cup
Bran muffin $-$ 1 (see recipe
page 140)
Margarine $-$ 1 tsp
Multivitamin $-$ 1

NOON MEAL

Fresh spinach salad
  Spinach $-$ 8 large leaves
  Mushrooms $-\frac{1}{2}$ cup
  Cherry tomatoes $-$ 6
  Green pepper and onion
  Crumbled bacon $-$ 1 tbs
  Low calorie salad
  dressing

Rye crackers $-$ 6 wafers
Mandarin oranges, canned
$-\frac{1}{2}$ cup

EVENING MEAL
(*opposite*)

Bean salad $-$ cold
  Kidney beans, cooked $-\frac{1}{2}$
  cup
  Onions, chopped $-\frac{1}{4}$ cup
  Garbanzo beans, cooked
  $-\frac{1}{4}$ cup
  Green beans, cooked $-\frac{1}{2}$
  cup
  Beets, cooked, sliced $-\frac{1}{2}$
  cup
  Vinegar $-$ 1 tsp
  Corn oil $-$ 1 tsp
  Garlic or onion powder
  and black pepper to taste

Grilled fish $-$ 6 oz
Brown rice $-\frac{1}{3}$ cup
Cabbage $-\frac{1}{2}$ cup
Honeydew melon $-$ 1 cup

SNACK

Bran muffin $-$ 1 (see recipe
page 140)
Margarine $-$ 1 tsp
Skim milk $-\frac{1}{2}$ cup
Apple $-$ 1 large

SATURDAY

BREAKFAST	Oatmeal surprise (serves 2)*
	  Oatmeal, uncooked – 1 cup
	  Orange juice – $\frac{1}{4}$ cup
	  Raisins – 2 tbs
	  Walnuts, chopped – 1 tbs
	  Orange peel, grated – 1 tsp
	  Skim milk – $\frac{1}{2}$ cup
		Whole wheat toast – 1 slice
		Margarine – 1 tsp
		Multivitamin – 1

NOON MEAL	Kidney bean and rice casserole**
	  Kidney beans, cooked – $\frac{1}{2}$ cup
	  Onion – $\frac{1}{2}$ cup
	  Green pepper – $\frac{1}{2}$ cup
	  Bay leaf – 1
	  Brown rice, cooked – $\frac{2}{3}$ cup
	  Broccoli – $\frac{1}{2}$ cup
		Whole wheat bread – 1 slice
		Margarine – 1 tsp

EVENING MEAL (*opposite*)	Filet mignon – 4 oz Baked potato – $\frac{1}{2}$ Green beans – $\frac{1}{2}$ cup Cauliflower – $\frac{1}{2}$ cup Beets – $\frac{1}{2}$ cup Whole wheat roll – 1	Fresh strawberries – 1 cup with whole milk – 2 oz
SNACK	Post Toasties® – $\frac{1}{2}$ cup Skim milk – $\frac{1}{2}$ cup Banana – $\frac{1}{2}$ Graham crackers – 2 squares	

* Cook oatmeal in your usual way but add raisins, walnuts and orange peel when you add oats to water. Add orange juice when oats are cooked and let sit for 3 minutes with lid on pan.

** Combine all ingredients except rice in sauce pan. Season with garlic, salt and pepper to taste. Heat until onions and green peppers are cooked. Serve over rice.

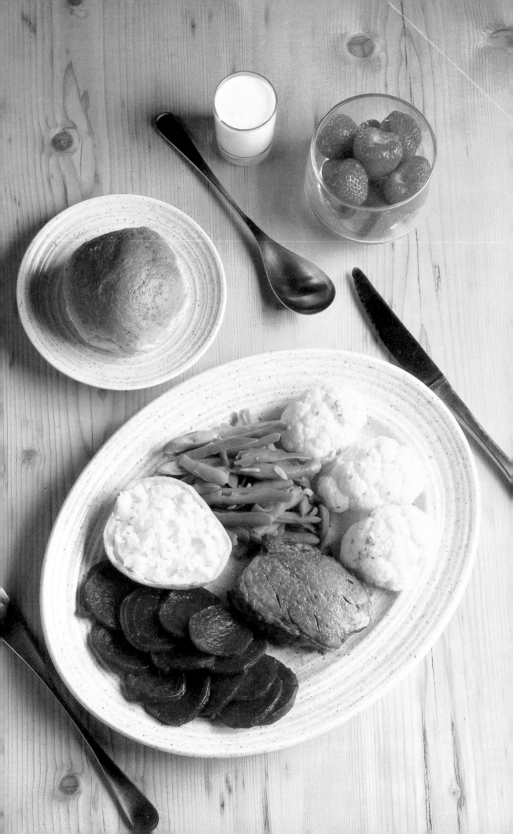

1200 CALORIE HIGH-FIBER MAINTENANCE DIET

This is suitable for many women over 50 who weigh between 100 and 120 lb (45 to 54 kg) or for overweight men weighing over 160 lb (72 kg) who are trying to lose weight.

SUNDAY

BREAKFAST
Corn flakes – 1 cup
Strawberries – $\frac{1}{2}$ cup
Skim milk – 8 oz
Pineapple juice – 4 oz
Multivitamin – 1

NOON MEAL
Dinner salad
Lettuce – 1 cup
Tomato – $\frac{1}{2}$
Cucumbers, radishes, green onion, celery, mushrooms
Low calorie dressing
Beef, lean – 4 oz
Green beans – 1 cup
Peaches, canned (unsweetened) – $\frac{1}{2}$ cup

EVENING MEAL
Stuffed green peppers
Green peppers – 2
Savory lentil rice – $1\frac{1}{2}$ cups (recipe listed for Saturday)
Carrots, cooked – $\frac{3}{4}$ cup
Beets, cold – $\frac{2}{3}$ cup
Whole wheat bread – 1 slice
Margarine – 1 tsp
Plums – 4

SNACK
Bran muffin – 1 (see recipe, page 140)
Margarine – 1 tsp
Pear – 1

MONDAY

BREAKFAST
Oatmeal – 1 cup with raisins (20)
Skim milk – 6 oz
Orange juice – 4 oz
Multivitamin – 1

NOON MEAL
Chef salad
Lettuce – 2 cups
Tomato – $\frac{1}{4}$
Radishes – 3
Cucumber – $\frac{1}{4}$
Green pepper – $\frac{1}{8}$
Zero dressing – 2 tbs
Whole wheat bread – 2 slices
Margarine – 1 tsp
Pineapple – $\frac{1}{2}$ cup

EVENING MEAL
Cod, broiled – 4 oz
Rice, brown – 1 cup
Corn – $\frac{2}{3}$ cup
Asparagus – $\frac{1}{2}$ cup
Bran muffin – 1 (see recipe page 140)
Margarine – 1 tsp
Fruit cocktail – $\frac{1}{2}$ cup

SNACK
Strawberries – 1 cup
Skim milk – 2 oz
Graham crackers – 2 squares

TUESDAY

BREAKFAST
Shredded Wheat® – 2 large
Skim milk – 8 oz
Grapefruit – $\frac{1}{2}$
Multivitamin – 1

NOON MEAL
Turkey sandwich
Light rye – 2 slices
Turkey – 2 oz
Lettuce – 3 leaves
Salad dressing – 1 tsp
Tomato – $\frac{1}{2}$
Melon – $\frac{1}{2}$ (muskmellon, honeydew or canteloupe)

EVENING MEAL
Navy beans – 1 cup
Ham – 2 oz
Onions – $\frac{1}{4}$ cup
Cornbread – 1 square
Cabbage – $\frac{3}{4}$ cup
Broccoli – $\frac{3}{4}$ cup
Peaches, canned – $\frac{1}{2}$ cup

SNACK
Grapes – 16
Rye crackers – 3

WEDNESDAY

BREAKFAST
Breakfast pattie (sausage substitute) – 1 oz
Hash brown potatoes – $\frac{2}{3}$ cup
Whole wheat toast – 1 slice
Orange – 1
Multivitamin – 1

NOON MEAL
Fresh spinach and mushroom salad
Spinach – 4 large leaves
Mushrooms – 6 medium
Bacon bits – 1 tsp
Low calorie dressing – 1 tbs
Rye crackers – 3
Pear – 1

EVENING MEAL
Roast beef – 3 oz
Brown rice – 1 cup
Lima beans – $\frac{1}{2}$ cup
Carrots, cooked – $\frac{3}{4}$ cup
Whole wheat dinner roll – 1
Plums – 4

SNACK
Grapenuts® – $\frac{1}{3}$ cup
Skim milk – 8 oz
Banana – $\frac{1}{2}$

THURSDAY	FRIDAY
BREAKFAST	**BREAKFAST**
Wheat flakes (Wheaties®) – 1 cup	Oatmeal – 1 cup
Skim milk – 6 oz	with banana – $\frac{1}{2}$
Orange juice – 4 oz	Skim milk – 8 oz
Multivitamin – 1	Multivitamin – 1
NOON MEAL	**NOON MEAL**
Ham sandwich	Cottage cheese – 1 cup
Lean ham – 1 oz	Cold beets – $\frac{2}{3}$ cup
Rye bread – 2 slices	Tomato – 1 medium
Lettuce – 3 slices	Cucumber – $\frac{1}{2}$ medium
Mustard	Peaches, canned – 1 cup
Carrots – 8 sticks	Rye crackers – 3
Celery – 3 sticks	
Plums – 4	
EVENING MEAL	**EVENING MEAL**
Spaghetti – 1 cup	Flounder – 4 oz
Meat sauce	Brown rice – 1 cup
Tomato sauce – 4 oz	Pinto beans – $\frac{1}{2}$ cup
Ground beef – 2 oz	Summer squash – $\frac{1}{2}$ cup
Corn – $\frac{2}{3}$ cup	Pumpernickel – 1 slice
Green beans – 1 cup	Margarine – 1 tsp
Rye bread – 1 slice	Apple sauce – $\frac{1}{2}$ cup
Margarine – 1 tsp	with cinnamon
Peaches, canned – $\frac{1}{2}$ cup	
SNACK	**SNACK**
Bran muffin – 1 (see recipe page 140)	Graham crackers – 4 squares
Strawberries – 1 cup	Pears, canned – 1 cup
Skim milk – 2 oz	

SATURDAY

BREAKFAST
Orange sections – $\frac{1}{2}$ cup
Breakfast pattie – 1
Spanish omelet
Egg whites – 2
Chopped green pepper,
pimento, onion, green
chili, tomato
Cheddar cheese – 1 oz
Whole wheat toast – 1 slice
Multivitamin – 1

NOON MEAL
Grapenut-fruit delight
Grapenuts® – $\frac{1}{3}$ cup
Yogurt – 5 oz
Peaches, canned – $\frac{1}{2}$ cup
Pears, canned – $\frac{1}{2}$ cup
Strawberries frozen – $\frac{1}{2}$
cup

EVENING MEAL
Savory lentil rice casserole
(see note page 117 for
cooking instructions)
Lentils, cooked – $\frac{1}{2}$ cup
Brown rice, cooked – 1
cup
Beef bouillon
Chopped onion – 1 tbs
Tomato juice – $\frac{1}{2}$ cup
Sweet basil – pinch
(optional)
Beets – $\frac{2}{3}$ cup
Broccoli – $\frac{2}{3}$ cup
Fruit cocktail – $\frac{1}{2}$ cup

SNACK
Turkey sandwich
Turkey – 1 oz
Rye bread – 2 slices
Lettuce – 3 leaves
Mayonnaise – 1 tsp
Grapes – 16

1600 CALORIE HIGH-FIBER DIET DESIGNED TO LOWER BLOOD CHOLESTEROL CONTENT

This diet would be suitable for some men weighing about 140 lb (64 kg) or for heavier individuals who wish to lose weight.

BREAKFAST	Oat bran cereal $-\frac{1}{4}$ cup (dry)* Skim milk – 1 cup Banana $-\frac{1}{2}$ Whole wheat toast – 2 slices Margarine – 1 tsp Multivitamin – 1

NOON MEAL	Cole slaw
	    Low calorie slaw dressing
	    Cabbage, finely shredded $-\frac{1}{2}$ cup
	    Celery seed and dill weed to taste
	Kidney bean and rice casserole (see Saturday, 1500 calorie diet, page 122)
	Oat muffin – 1**
	Margarine – 1 tsp
	Apple – 1 medium

EVENING MEAL	Dinner salad (see Sunday, 1500 calorie diet, page 111) Roast turkey – 4 oz Potatoes, mashed $-\frac{1}{2}$ cup Green beans $-\frac{1}{2}$ cup Oat muffin – 1 Margarine – 1 tsp Peaches, canned $-\frac{1}{2}$ cup
SNACK	Whole wheat bread – 2 slices Margarine – 1 tsp Tangerine – 1

* Cook as directed on box. Use oat meal if oat bran is unavailable in your area.

** Add $\frac{1}{4}$ cup egg substitute (2 egg whites or Eggbeaters®) to mixing bowl and beat well. Pour 1 cup of skim milk into bowl and mix. In a separate bowl mix well 1 cup self-raising flour, 1 cup oat bran and 1 tsp cinnamon. Mix dry and liquid ingredients together until well blended. Do not beat. Dice $\frac{1}{2}$ pear (canned) and add to mixture. Spray muffin pan with Pam® and add mix. Bake at 400°F for 15 minutes. (Makes 10 to 12 muffins.)

1500 CALORIE HIGH-FIBER DIET DESIGNED TO TREAT HYPOGLYCEMIA

This diet is appropriate for some young middle-aged individuals weighing between 115 and 130 lb (52 and 59 kg).

BREAKFAST	Oatmeal, dry $-\frac{1}{4}$ cup Skim milk $-\frac{1}{3}$ cup Banana $-\frac{1}{2}$ Whole wheat toast $-$ 1 slice Margarine $-$ 1 tsp Multivitamin $-$ 1
SNACK	Graham crackers $-$ 2 squares

NOON MEAL	Sprout salad (see Wednesday, 1500 calorie diet, page 117)
	Turkey sandwich
	   Whole wheat bread $-$ 2 slices
	   Turkey $-$ 1$\frac{1}{2}$ oz
	   Mayonnaise $-$ 1 tsp
	   Lettuce $-$ 5 leaves
	Tomato $-$ 1 small
	Apple $-$ 1 medium

SNACK	Grapenuts® $-$ 3 tbs Skim milk $-\frac{1}{3}$ cup
EVENING MEAL	Broiled fish $-$ 5 oz Brown rice $-\frac{2}{3}$ cup Corn $-\frac{1}{2}$ cup Carrots $-\frac{1}{2}$ cup Bran muffin $-$ 1 (see recipe page 140) Margarine $-$ 2 tsp Peaches, canned $-\frac{1}{2}$ cup
SNACK	Corn flakes $-$ 1 cup Skim milk $-\frac{1}{3}$ cup Rye wafers $-$ 3 Margarine $-$ 1 tsp

Guide to food exchanges

MILK EXCHANGES

One exchange averages:

11 grams carbohydrate
8 grams protein
0.5 gram fat
0 grams fiber
80 calories

Skim milk	1 cup
Skim milk, powdered	3 tbs
Skim milk, evaporated	$\frac{1}{2}$ cup
Yogurt, skim, plain	5 oz
Yogurt, 2% fat, plain	4 oz

A VEGETABLE EXCHANGES
(Low calorie vegetables)

One exchange averages:

2 grams carbohydrate
1 gram protein
0 grams fat
2 grams fiber
13 calories

Bean sprouts	$\frac{1}{2}$ cup
Beans, green, raw	$\frac{1}{2}$ cup
Beans, runner, raw	$\frac{1}{2}$ cup
Beans, string, raw	$\frac{1}{2}$ cup
Cabbage, cooked	$\frac{1}{2}$ cup
Cabbage, red or white	$\frac{1}{2}$ cup
Carrots, cooked	$\frac{1}{2}$ cup
Carrots, raw, grated	$\frac{1}{2}$ cup
Cauliflower, cooked	$\frac{1}{2}$ cup
Cauliflower, raw	$\frac{1}{2}$ cup
Eggplant, raw	$\frac{1}{2}$ cup
Kale, cooked	$\frac{1}{2}$ cup
Okra, raw	$\frac{1}{2}$ cup
Onion, cooked	$\frac{1}{2}$ cup
Onion, raw	$\frac{1}{2}$ cup
Onion, spring, raw	2 medium
Pepper, green, raw	$\frac{1}{2}$ cup
Squash, summer, cooked	$\frac{1}{2}$ cup
Turnip greens, cooked	$\frac{1}{2}$ cup

Free vegetables

You may have $\frac{1}{2}$ to 1 cup of the following raw vegetables per meal.

Celery
Cress greens
Cucumbers
Lettuce
Mushrooms

Mustard greens
Radishes
Spinach
Zucchini

B VEGETABLE EXCHANGES

One exchange averages:

4 grams carbohydrate
2 grams protein
0 grams fat
2 grams fiber
24 calories

Beets, cooked	$\frac{1}{2}$ cup
Beets, raw	$\frac{1}{2}$ cup
Brussels sprouts, cooked	$\frac{1}{2}$ cup
Brussels sprouts, raw	$\frac{1}{2}$ cup
Kale, raw	1 cup
Rutabaga, raw	$\frac{1}{2}$ cup
Spinach, cooked	$\frac{1}{2}$ cup
Tomatoes, cooked	$\frac{1}{2}$ cup
Tomatoes, raw	1 small

C VEGETABLE EXCHANGES
(Starchy vegetables)

One exchange averages:

15 grams carbohydrate
2 grams protein
0.5 gram fat
3 grams fiber
75 calories

Barley, pearled, dry	$1\frac{1}{2}$ tbs
Corn, sweet, cooked	$\frac{1}{2}$ cup
Corn, sweet, raw	$\frac{1}{2}$ medium ear
Peas, processed, raw	$\frac{1}{2}$ cup
Potatoes, sweet, baked	$\frac{1}{2}$ medium
Potatoes, white, baked	$\frac{1}{2}$ medium
Potatoes, white, cooked	$\frac{1}{2}$ cup
Rice, brown, cooked	$\frac{1}{3}$ cup
Rice, white, cooked	$\frac{1}{3}$ cup
Squash, winter, cooked	1 cup
Yams, cooked (with skins)	$\frac{1}{3}$ cup

BEAN EXCHANGES

One exchange averages:

12.5 grams carbohydrate
6.5 grams protein
0.5 gram fat
8 grams fiber
80 calories

Beans, brown, cooked	$\frac{1}{2}$ cup
Beans, kidney, cooked	$\frac{1}{2}$ cup
Beans, lima, cooked	$\frac{1}{2}$ cup
Beans, pinto, cooked	$\frac{1}{2}$ cup
Beans, white, cooked	$\frac{1}{2}$ cup
Lentils, cooked	$\frac{1}{2}$ cup

CEREAL EXCHANGES

One exchange averages:

13 grams carbohydrate
2.5 grams protein
0.5 gram fat
3 grams fiber
70 calories

All Bran®	$\frac{1}{3}$ cup
Bran Chex®	$\frac{1}{2}$ cup
Corn Chex®	$\frac{3}{4}$ cup
Corn Bran®	$\frac{1}{2}$ cup
Corn Flakes®	$\frac{3}{4}$ cup
Grapenut Flakes®	$\frac{2}{3}$ cup
Grapenuts®	3 tbs
Grits, dry	2 tbs
Oat bran, dry	$\frac{1}{4}$ cup
Fortified Oat Flakes®	$\frac{1}{2}$ cup
Oatmeal, instant, dry	$\frac{3}{4}$ package
Oats, whole, dry	$\frac{1}{4}$ cup
100% Bran®	$\frac{1}{3}$ cup
Post Toasties®	1 cup
Puffed Wheat®	$\frac{3}{4}$ cup
Ralston®, dry	3 tbs
Shredded Wheat®	1 biscuit
Total®	$\frac{3}{4}$ cup
Wheaties®	$\frac{3}{4}$ cup

OPPOSITE AND OVERLEAF: The four pages that follow show a tempting selection of vegetables, beans, fruit and meat.

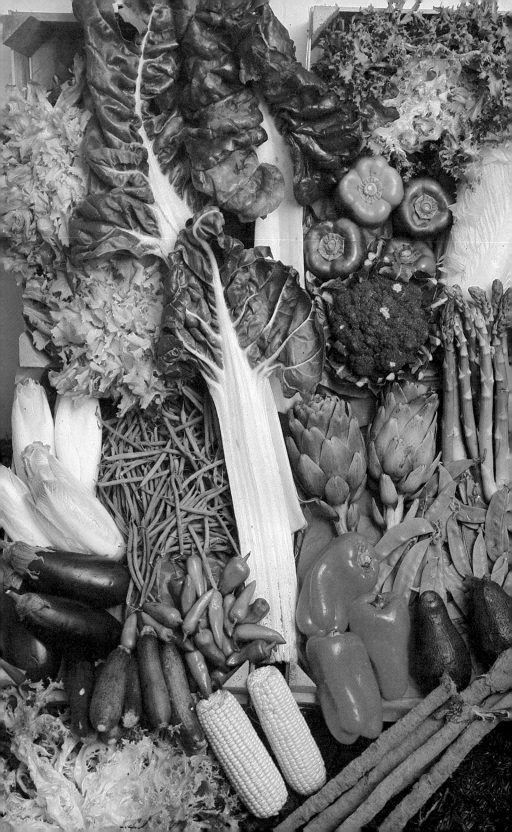

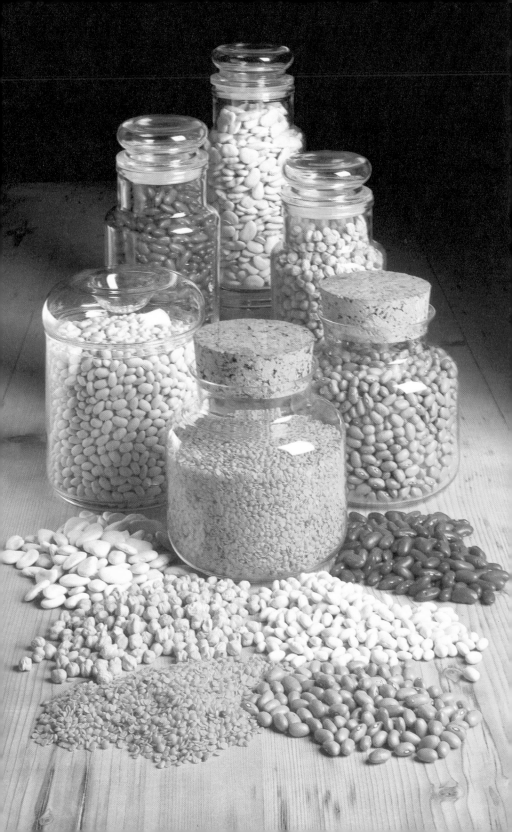

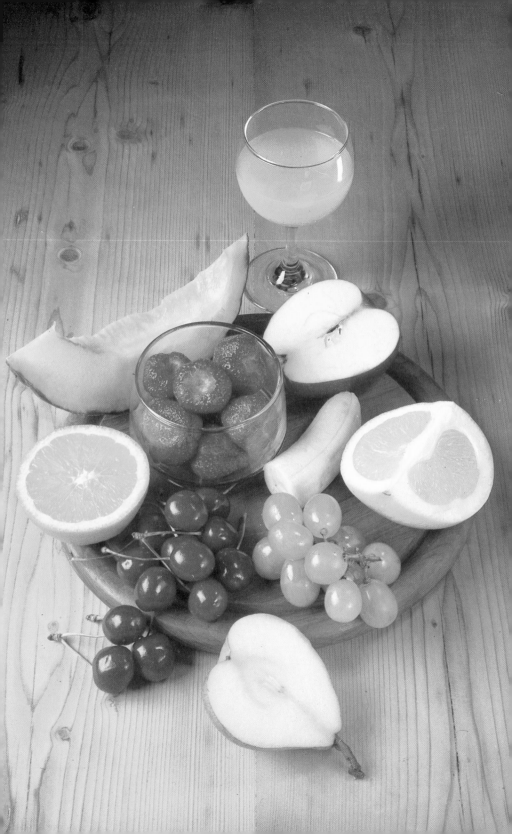

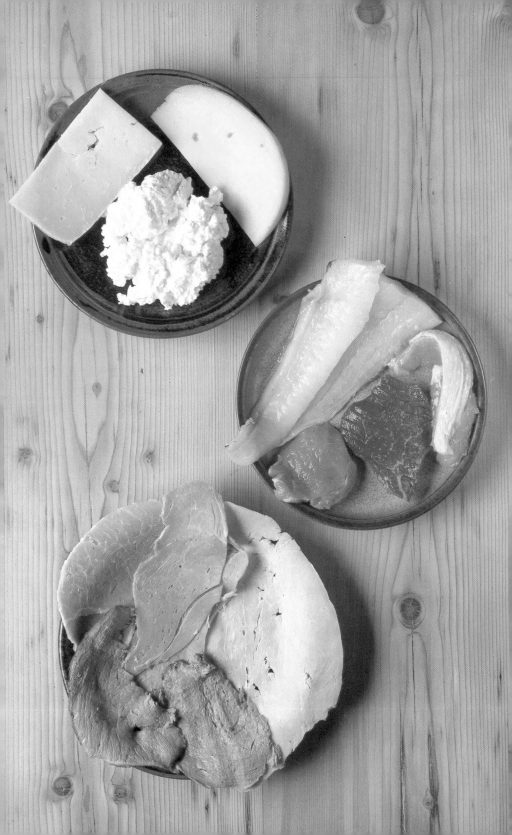

BREAD EXCHANGES

One exchange averages:

11 grams carbohydrate
2 grams protein
0.5 gram fat
2 grams fiber
60 calories

Bread, pumpernickel	$\frac{3}{4}$ slice
Bread, rye	1 slice
Bread, whole meal wheat	1 slice
Bread, whole wheat	1 slice
Cornmeal, degerminated, yellow	2 tbs
Cracker, Graham	2 squares
Cracker, rye	3 wafers
Cracker, whole wheat	6 crackers
Flour, oat, whole grain	$2\frac{1}{2}$ tbs
Flour, rye, dark	$2\frac{1}{2}$ tbs
Flour, rye, light	$2\frac{1}{2}$ tbs
Flour, whole meal (100%) wheat	$2\frac{1}{2}$ tbs
Flour, whole wheat (85%)	$2\frac{1}{2}$ tbs
Macaroni, whole wheat, cooked	$\frac{1}{2}$ cup
Muffin, whole wheat	1
Popcorn, popped	3 cups
Roll, whole wheat	$\frac{3}{4}$ roll
Spaghetti, whole wheat (cooked)	$\frac{1}{2}$ cup
Wheat bran	$\frac{1}{2}$ cup

FRUIT EXCHANGES

One exchange averages:

10 grams carbohydrate
0 grams protein
0 grams fat
2 grams fiber
40 calories

Apple, raw	$\frac{1}{2}$ large
Apple, cooked	$\frac{1}{2}$ large
Apple sauce, C.U.*	$\frac{1}{3}$ cup
Apple juice, C.U.	$\frac{1}{3}$ cup
Apricots, raw	2
Apricots, C.U.	$\frac{1}{4}$ cup
Banana, fresh	$\frac{1}{2}$ medium
Blackberries, raw	$\frac{3}{4}$ cup
Cantaloupe	1 cup
Cherries, raw	10 large
Cherries, cooked	$\frac{1}{2}$ cup
Cherries, C.U.	$\frac{1}{3}$ cup
Cranberries, raw	$\frac{1}{2}$ cup
Dates, dried	2

Figs, dried	1 medium
Grapes, black	15
Grapes, white	10
Grape juice, C.U.	$\frac{1}{4}$ cup
Grapefruit, raw	$\frac{1}{2}$
Grapefruit, C.U.	$\frac{1}{2}$ cup
Honeydew melon	1 cup
Nectarine, raw	1 small
Orange, raw	1 small
Orange juice, C.U.	$\frac{1}{3}$ cup
Oranges, mandarin, C.U.	$\frac{1}{2}$ cup
Peach, raw	1 medium
Peaches, C.U.	$\frac{1}{4}$ cup
Pear, raw	$\frac{1}{2}$ medium
Pears, C.U.	$\frac{1}{4}$ cup
Pineapple, raw	$\frac{1}{2}$ cup
Pineapple juice, C.U.	$\frac{1}{3}$ cup
Plums, raw	3 small
Plums, C.U.	$\frac{1}{3}$ cup
Prunes, dried	2
Prunes, C.U.	2 medium
Raisins, dried	$1\frac{1}{2}$ tbs
Raspberries, red, raw	1 cup
Raspberries, red, C.U.	$\frac{1}{2}$ cup
Strawberries, raw	1 cup
Tangerine, raw	1 large
Watermelon	1 cup

* C.U. – canned, unsweetened

MEAT EXCHANGES

One exchange averages:	
	0 grams carbohydrate
	8 grams protein
	2 grams fat
	0 grams fiber
	50 calories

Beef, rump or tenderloin	1 oz
Cheese, cottage, low fat	$\frac{1}{2}$ cup
Cheese, cottage, creamed	$\frac{1}{4}$ cup
Cheese, countdown	1 oz
Cheese, mozzarella	$\frac{3}{4}$ oz
Cheese, ricotta	$1\frac{1}{2}$ oz
Chicken, dark	1 oz
Chicken, light	1 oz
Duck, raw	1 oz
Egg substitutes	$\frac{1}{4}$ cup
Egg white	3 large
Fish, bass	2 oz
catfish	2 oz
cod	2 oz

flounder	2 oz
haddock	2 oz
halibut	2 oz
ocean perch	2 oz
red snapper	2 oz
salmon	1 oz
sardines, water packed	5 small
sole	2 oz
trout	2 oz
tuna, water packed	$\frac{1}{4}$ cup
Goose, raw	1 oz
Lamb, leg or loin	1 oz
Pork, ham or lean	1 oz
Pork, loin, picnic	1 oz
Turkey, dark	1 oz
Turkey, light	1 oz

FAT EXCHANGES

One exchange averages:

1 gram carbohydrate
0 grams protein
4.5 grams fat
0 grams fiber
45 calories

Dressings

French	2 tsp
French, low fat	2 tbs
Salad (mayonnaise type)	2 tsp
1000 Island	2 tsp
1000 Island, low fat	2 tbs

Margarine

Bar	1 tsp
Liquid	1 tsp
Tub	2 tsp

Mayonnaise

Safflower and soy oil	1 tsp
Soybean oil type	1 tsp

Nuts

Almonds, whole	1 tbs
Chestnuts	3
Peanuts, roasted	1 tbs
Pecans	1 tbs

Oils

Corn	1 tsp
Safflower	1 tsp
Soybean	1 tsp
Wheatgerm	1 tsp

WHOLE WHEAT BRAN MUFFINS

White flour	1 cup
Whole meal flour	1 cup
All Bran®	$\frac{1}{2}$ cup
Baking powder	1 tsp
Liquid artificial sweetener	$\frac{1}{2}$ tsp
Skim milk	$\frac{1}{2}$ cup
Egg white	1 large
Corn oil	1 tbs

Slightly beat egg white with a fork. Add milk, corn oil and artificial sweetener.

Mix dry ingredients well. Pour milk mixture into dry ingredients, mix with fork. Don't overmix.

Oil muffin pans (or 8 in×8 in baking tin) lightly (or spray with Pam®).

Pour in batter and bake at 375°F for 20 minutes. Divide into 12 portions.

1 muffin=2 bread exchanges

CORNBREAD

Self-raising flour	1 cup
Yellow or white cornmeal	$\frac{1}{3}$ cup
Skim milk	1 cup
Egg white	1 large

Slightly beat egg white with a fork. Add milk and mix well.

Measure flour and cornmeal and mix well. Add liquid to dry ingredients. Mix briefly with a fork.

Oil muffin pans (or 8 in×8 in baking tin) lightly (or spray with Pam®).

Bake at 400°F for 15 to 20 minutes until golden brown. Divide into 12 pieces.

1 piece=2 bread exchanges

Guide to fiber in foods

Food	Serving size	Grams/ serving	Calories/ serving	Fiber, in grams/ serving
Apple, fresh	$\frac{1}{2}$ large	83	42	2.0
Apple, cooked	$\frac{1}{2}$ large	83	40	2.0
Apricots, fresh	2	72	32	1.4
Asparagus, cooked	$\frac{1}{2}$ cup	93	18	3.5
Banana, fresh	$\frac{1}{2}$ medium	54	48	1.5
Bean sprouts, fresh	$\frac{1}{2}$ cup	58	13	1.5
Beans, brown, cooked	$\frac{1}{2}$ cup	84	80	8.4
Beans, green, cooked	$\frac{1}{2}$ cup	64	10	2.1
Beans, kidney, cooked	$\frac{1}{2}$ cup	93	94	9.7
Beans, lima, cooked	$\frac{1}{2}$ cup	85	63	8.3
Beans, pinto, cooked	$\frac{1}{2}$ cup	84	78	8.9
Beans, white, cooked	$\frac{1}{2}$ cup	90	79	7.9
Beets, cooked	$\frac{1}{2}$ cup	85	33	2.1
Blackberries, fresh	$\frac{3}{4}$ cup	108	40	6.7
Bread, pumpernickel	$\frac{3}{4}$ slice	24	58	1.4
cornbread	1 square	30	58	1.1
French	1 slice	25	71	0.7
rye	1 slice	25	62	0.8
white	1 slice	25	64	0.7
whole meal	1 slice	25	56	2.1
whole wheat	1 slice	25	59	1.3
Broccoli, cooked	$\frac{1}{2}$ cup	93	18	3.5
Brussels sprouts, cooked	$\frac{1}{2}$ cup	78	20	2.3
Cabbage, white, cooked	$\frac{1}{2}$ cup	85	10	2.1
Carrots, raw	$\frac{1}{2}$ cup	55	15	1.8
Cauliflower, cooked	$\frac{1}{2}$ cup	90	14	1.6
Celery, raw	$\frac{1}{2}$ cup	60	8	1.1
Cereal, All Bran® (100%)	$\frac{1}{3}$ cup	28	70	8.4
Bran Chex®	$\frac{1}{2}$ cup	21	67	4.1
Corn Chex®	$\frac{3}{4}$ cup	21	71	2.6
Corn Bran®	$\frac{1}{2}$ cup	21	68	4.4
Corn Flakes®	$\frac{3}{4}$ cup	21	70	2.6
Grapenut Flakes®	$\frac{2}{3}$ cup	21	71	2.5
Grapenuts®	3 tbs	21	70	2.7
Oat Bran®, dry	$\frac{1}{4}$ cup	20	58	5.3
Oat Flakes	$\frac{1}{2}$ cup	21	72	2.5
Oatmeal, instant dry	$\frac{3}{4}$ pkg	21	74	2.5
Oats, whole dry	$\frac{1}{4}$ cup	21	71	2.9
Post Toasties®	1 cup	21	71	2.6
Puffed Wheat®	$\frac{3}{4}$ cup	21	68	3.4
Ralston® dry	3 tbs	21	72	2.1
Shredded Wheat®	1 biscuit	21	70	2.8
Total®	$\frac{3}{4}$ cup	21	75	2.5
Wheaties®	$\frac{3}{4}$ cup	14	73	2.6
Cherries, fresh	10 large	68	38	1.1
Corn, sweet, fresh	$\frac{1}{2}$ med. ear	63	72	2.6
Cornmeal, fine	2 tbs	17	57	1.6

Food	Serving size	Grams/ serving	Calories/ serving	Fiber, in grams/ serving
Cracker, graham	2 squares	14	53	1.4
rye wafer	3 wafers	20	64	2.3
saltine	6 crackers	20	76	0.8
Cranberries, raw	½ cup	96	31	4.0
Cucumber, raw	½ cup	70	6	1.1
Eggplant, raw	½ cup	100	16	2.5
Figs, dried	1 medium	20	46	3.7
Flour, rye, dark	2½ tbs	20	63	2.5
rye, light	2½ tbs	16	56	0.5
self-raising	2½ tbs	18	61	0.7
wheat, white	2½ tbs	18	62	0.5
wheat, whole meal	2½ tbs	19	60	1.8
wheat, whole wheat	2½ tbs	19	62	1.4
Grapefruit, fresh	½	87	31	0.8
Grapes, black, fresh	15	60	45	0.5
Grapes, white, fresh	10	50	36	0.5
Kale, cooked	½ cup	65	15	1.3
Lentils, cooked	½ cup	100	97	3.7
Lettuce, fresh	1 cup	55	5	0.8
Macaroni, cooked	½ cup	70	77	0.6
Melon, cantaloupe	1 cup	160	39	1.6
honeydew	1 cup	170	42	1.5
watermelon	1 cup	160	35	1.4
Mushrooms, raw	½ cup	35	7	0.9
Mustard greens, raw	1 cup	55	7	2.0
Nectarine, raw	1 small	69	44	1.5
Nuts, almonds, whole	1 tbs	8	46	1.1
chestnuts	3	26	46	1.8
peanuts, roasted	1 tbs	9	52	0.8
pecans	1 tbs	7.5	49	0.5
Okra, raw	½ cup	50	13	1.6
Onion, raw	½ cup	58	14	1.2
Orange, fresh	1 small	78	35	1.6
Peach, fresh	1 medium	100	38	2.3
Pear, fresh	½ medium	82	44	2.0
Peas, canned, cooked	½ cup	85	63	6.7
Pepper, green, raw	½ cup	58	10	1.1
Pineapple, fresh	½ cup	78	41	0.8
Plum, fresh	3 small	85	38	1.8
Popcorn, popped	3 cups	18	62	3.0
Potato, sweet, cooked	½ medium	75	79	2.1
Potato, white, baked	½ medium	75	72	1.9
Prunes, dried	2	15	38	2.8
Radishes, raw	½ cup	58	7	1.3
Raisins, dried	1½ tbs	14	39	1.0
Raspberries, red, fresh	1 cup	124	42	9.2
Rice, brown, cooked	⅓ cup	65	72	1.6
Rice, white, cooked	⅓ cup	68	76	0.5
Roll, dinner	¾ roll	20	60	0.6
Roll, whole wheat	¾ roll	21	55	1.2

Food	Serving size	Grams/ serving	Calories/ serving	Fiber, in grams/ serving
Spaghetti, cooked	$\frac{1}{2}$ cup	70	76	0.8
Spinach, fresh	1 cup	55	8	0.2
Squash, summer, cooked	$\frac{1}{2}$ cup	90	8	2.0
Squash, winter, cooked	1 cup	240	82	7.0
Strawberries, fresh	1 cup	143	45	3.1
Tangerine, fresh	1 large	101	39	2.0
Tomato, cooked	$\frac{1}{2}$ cup	121	20	1.5
Tomato, raw	1 small	100	18	1.5
Turnip, cooked	$\frac{1}{2}$ cup	93	12	2.0
Yam, cooked	$\frac{1}{3}$ cup	66	72	2.6
Zucchini, raw	$\frac{1}{2}$ cup	65	7	2.0

10 NEW DEVELOPMENTS IN DIABETES RESEARCH

During the next few years we shall be seeing more pancreas transplants, artificial pancreases, practical methods for measuring the blood sugar at home, manufacture of human insulin, and many improvements in the control of diabetes. We are on the threshold of many more breakthroughs and new discoveries. Some of this new knowledge is already being used to treat diabetics; many more novel approaches will be used to improve the lifestyle of diabetic patients. In this chapter, I want to give you an overview of some of these new developments and my predictions about their future use.

The artificial pancreas

The artificial pancreas has three parts. A glucose sensor measures the blood sugar continuously, a computer makes decisions about how much insulin to give, and a pump automatically injects the correct amount of insulin. The artificial pancreas has been available since about 1975. Unfortunately this machine is about the size of a washing machine . . . certainly not portable!

Several centers are working on small glucose sensors to measure the blood sugar. When experiments were made using the sensors placed in animals, they had a tendency to get plugged with proteins from the blood. Nevertheless, a glucose sensor about the size of a coin (3 cm or 1 inch across and 5 mm or $\frac{1}{4}$ inch thick) may soon be available. The computer will not be a major problem once the sensor and pump have been developed. Current pumps are about the size of a pack of cigarettes. It's likely that a complete artificial pancreas, to be placed under the skin of the abdomen or chest and refilled with insulin daily or weekly, will be available within five years.

Insulin infusion pumps

These are now being used all over the world, but they serve only the third function of an artificial pancreas. Currently, patients measure their blood

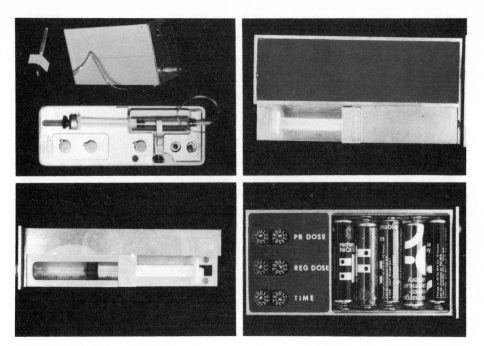

Two insulin infusion pumps.

sugars three to eight times daily – this is the glucose sensor. Then, with the guidance of their doctor, they decide how much insulin the pump should give – the patient's brain is the computer. These insulin infusion pumps have been used in several medical centers since 1977, but there are still some problems with them.

Most insulin pumps are worn in a holster attached to a belt. Insulin is pumped from a reservoir through a small plastic tube into the subcutaneous tissues lying under the skin. Usually insulin is given into the subcutaneous tissue of the abdomen but may be given in the arms or legs. Most patients receive a slow and continuous infusion of insulin at a 'basal rate', which regulates the blood sugar between meals. Before the three major meals, and sometimes before snacks, additional insulin is given. By pushing a button a pre-meal 'pulse' of insulin is given, which may range from 5 to 30 units of regular insulin before each meal. All these insulin doses have to be carefully worked out by the medical team.

What are the disadvantages of insulin infusion pumps?
Available pumps are large and bulky, about 25 cm (10 in) long, 8 cm (3 in) wide and 3 cm (1 in) thick. A leather belt and holster do not go well with evening dress, a dressy men's suit, a swimsuit or other clothes. Current pumps are not as convenient and safe as they should be. Pumps must be

designed which cannot – I repeat – cannot deliver more insulin than intended. Shortly, pumps even smaller than a pack of cigarettes, with these safety features, will be available.

The injection of insulin into the subcutaneous tissue has disadvantages. Insulin is absorbed slowly, and at an unpredictable rate, from this area. Some people rapidly destroy insulin that is given into the subcutaneous tissue, so they must have injection through the veins. Some medical centers are testing the delivery of insulin into the large veins close to the heart (the superior vena cava). Insulin is pumped through a small rubber tube which enters the skin above the breast and travels under the skin into the neck and then through veins into the superior vena cava. This approach has many advantages. First, the tubing is not changed very often; some patients have had tubes like this for eight years. Second, the absorption of insulin is predictable, and insulin is not destroyed in the subcutaneous tissue. Third, when insulin is given by vein it acts much more quickly and more predictably than from the subcutaneous tissue. So, injected insulin can act more like insulin from the pancreas. However, further studies are needed to determine the suitability of insulin infusions direct into the veins (intravenous) and into the abdominal cavity (intraperitoneal).

What is the future role of insulin infusion pumps?
These pumps will be very popular as most patients can achieve good or excellent blood sugar values with them. After the patient and the physician realize that good or excellent control is achievable, other avenues can be explored. Most patients can control their blood sugar as well with three or four injections of insulin per day as with a pump, so they will elect to take their daily injections and not be bothered by a mechanical device. However, some patients may use the pump during the sleeping hours (9 pm to 7 am) to maintain a good supply of insulin through the night.

Some patients will benefit from long-term insulin infusions into a large vein. Overall, these insulin pumps represent a major breakthrough in the treatment of diabetes. They have demonstrated that even difficult-to-control diabetes can be managed by the appropriate delivery of insulin.

Pancreas transplants

Diabetes can be cured by a pancreas transplant. Unfortunately, only a few medical centers do pancreas transplants, and there are many more failures than successes. One total success, however, is all that is required to prove that a pancreas transplant is worthwhile. There have been several long-term successes, so these transplants will be available for highly selected patients in this decade. I will briefly describe some problems, and several approaches that have been used.

Why are pancreas transplants so difficult?

The pancreas is primarily a factory. Most of its cells make digestive enzymes which help us break down proteins, fats and starches so their small components can be absorbed by the intestine. Diabetics, of course, have normal amounts of digestive enzymes and do not need this part of the pancreas. These enzymes are the major problem with transplantation.

First, they have to be drained from the pancreas so they do not damage the bed into which the pancreas transplant is laid. Second, the islands of the pancreas, known as the islets of Langerhans are widely scattered and amount to only 2 per cent of the total pancreas. The ideal procedure would be to separate out the islets and do an islet transplant, but this is very difficult to do. Third, when any tissue from another person (the donor) is transplanted into a recipient, the latter develops a protective response. The body fights infection by developing an immune response to destroy the invading infectious agent. In a similar way, the body of the recipient develops a vigorous immune response to destroy the 'foreign' tissue from the donor. Once the pancreas or islet transplant has been done successfully, the medical team must work diligently to prevent the recipient from destroying the new 'foreign' material. A variety of antirejection drugs, such as steroids and drugs which suppress the immune response, are given to prevent this destructive process and fight inflammation.

How are pancreas transplants done?

Early pioneers attempted to remove the entire pancreas from a donor and connect it with the diabetic recipient. This was extremely difficult to do and not very successful. All donors have been non-diabetic individuals who have died from some other cause. The pancreas must be removed immediately after death and transplanted as quickly as possible into the diabetic recipient. Currently, only a segment is transplanted.

Several techniques have been used to get rid of the troublesome digestive enzymes. First, a number of patients have had kidney transplants followed by pancreas transplants. These patients had developed severe kidney damage from their diabetes and as a result had to be given kidney transplants, so the digestive enzymes could be drained out of the body through the drainage system of the damaged kidney. The drainage tube of the pancreas (the pancreatic duct) is connected to the drainage tube (ureter) of the kidney. Second, the donor's pancreas can be connected to the intestine of the recipient and the digestive enzymes drained into the intestine; the normal way for them to enter the body. Unfortunately, this procedure is more difficult and complications are more likely when the intestine of the recipient is cut open. Third, the pancreas segment can be transplanted into the peritoneal cavity and the digestive enzymes released into it. This is a new technique which requires further study. All patients who receive pancreas transplants require large doses of antirejection drugs to prevent the recipient from destroying the donor pancreas.

How are islet transplants done?

Islet transplants have been very successful for curing diabetes in rats but not so far for people. The advantages of islet transplants are that: there are no digestive enzymes to worry about; the operation is very simple; antirejection drugs may not be required. But unfortunately there are several major obstacles. The procedure for isolating or harvesting islets from the pancreas is difficult. The digestive enzymes of the pancreas will digest the islets unless the procedure is done properly. Because of the difficulties in harvesting islets, adequate numbers of them cannot be taken from a single donor to cure diabetes in a recipient.

Fetal islets   Because of inadequate numbers of islets available, techniques are being developed to store them. Freezing the islets, known as cryopreservation, is satisfactory, but about half are destroyed during the freezing and thawing procedures. The newer tissue culture techniques, using islets from fetuses, have several advantages. After a miscarriage, abortion, or death of a premature infant, the islets of the fetus can be removed and placed in a culture media that supports growth and multiplication. Thus, a few thousand islet cells may yield much greater numbers. These islets are being preserved ready for islet transplants.

There are several advantages of transplants using fetal islets. First, there are no digestive enzymes to be drained. Second, the islets may not be regarded as foreign tissue by the recipient's body, as these fetal islets are immature cells without the adult features which alarm the body and cause an immune response. Large doses of antirejection drugs which have serious side-effects may therefore not be required. Third, the operation is very simple. Sometimes the islets are injected into the peritoneal cavity and the patient does not even have an incision. Sometimes they are injected into the portal vein (the large vein leading from the intestines to the liver) which is a very brief operation and requires only a small incision.

What is the future of pancreas transplants?
Transplants offer the only hope of cure for patients who already have diabetes. Even with currently available techniques, we cannot adequately control the blood sugar in many patients. Islet transplants will be a great blessing for many children with juvenile-type diabetes. I think that islet transplants using fetal islets have enormous potential, that suitable techniques for isolating and preserving the islets can be developed, and that this procedure will be a great benefit for selected patients. Pancreas transplants, now being done successfully, will continue to cure diabetes for a very limited number of selected patients.

Preventing diabetes

The ultimate goal, of course, is to prevent diabetes from actually developing. Ten years ago this only was an idle dream; now we have the tools to allow us to identify children who are likely to develop diabetes, and we are on the threshold of discovering techniques for this.

Identifying children with a tendency to be diabetic
The first step is to identify children who have a high likelihood of developing diabetes. As mentioned in chapter one, the inheritance patterns for diabetes are not consistent enough to predict which people have strong diabetic tendencies. New techniques such as special tissue typing must be developed to identify children at high risk.

Tissue typing at present is done before blood transfusions. You have A, B, AB, or O type blood and are either Rhesus (called Rh) positive or negative. My blood type for example, is O negative; this means that my blood can be given to another person with the same blood group and they will not have a blood transfusion reaction. The tissue type of white blood cells (leukocytes) can be measured, and this system is called the human leukocyte-A (HLA) system, through which hundreds of different tissue types can be recognized.

Recent research indicates that most children with the juvenile-type of diabetes have the same HLA tissue type. Further work is necessary to confirm and extend these observations. Nevertheless, before too long we may be able to measure a particular child's tissue type and tell whether he or she has a high or low probability of developing juvenile-type diabetes.

Preventing diabetes in susceptible children
If children who have a high risk of developing juvenile-type diabetes can be identified, two approaches may be used to prevent the disease. First, a

vaccine could be developed against a virus which causes diabetes. For example polio, once a major health problem, no longer develops in people who have had polio vaccines. If a virus or several viruses are responsible for the development of juvenile-type diabetes, vaccines might protect susceptible children from these viruses.

Second, a blocking antibody might be produced which protects the pancreas from damage. Before I explain this exciting possibility, I should tell you a little more about antibodies and their role in diabetes. We make antibodies to protect ourselves from 'foreign' invaders called antigens. After we have the measles for example, we develop special proteins called antibodies which prevent the measles virus from repeating as an infection. Thus, we are immune to measles. Children can be immunized against measles and develop the protective antibodies without having the infection. Children who develop juvenile-type diabetes have a problem in that the surface of their beta-cells (the islet cells of the pancreas which make insulin) has a protruding antigen. This is not a foreign antigen but a normal body protein. However, for unknown reasons, these children develop antibodies against their own insulin-making cells. This appears to be the basic cause of juvenile-type diabetes.

So can these children be protected from this tendency to destroy their own insulin-producing cells? If the antigen can be identified, then it may be possible to immunize these children in such a way that they would be protected from their own antibodies. As an example, mothers who had Rh-negative blood types used to develop antibodies against their own fetuses who had Rh-positive blood types. The newborn child developed severe jaundice because its mother's antibodies were destroying the child's red blood cells. This problem has now been solved, and with proper treatment, mothers do not develop antibodies and their children are not endangered by jaundice. In a somewhat analogous fashion, research scientists may be able to develop techniques to protect children from developing diabetes. The blocking antibody for example, may sit on the insulin-producing cell and protect it from other antibodies. In this way diabetes could be prevented.

11 CONCLUSION

The diabetic's motto should be 'happiness is knowing that your blood sugar is on target'. The vast majority of diabetics can keep their blood sugar on target by following the principles outlined in this book.

1. If you have adult-type diabetes which can be controlled by diet, you can keep your blood sugar within acceptable ranges by following a diet closely, watching your weight and regular exercise.

2. If you take oral hypoglycemic antidiabetes pills you also can maintain satisfactory blood sugar readings by following a good diabetic diet such as the HCF diet, maintaining a lean body weight, and taking appropriate exercise.

3. If you are overweight and take insulin, the chances are very good that you could stop your daily injections by losing weight and exercising regularly.

4. If you are lean, developed your diabetes after the age of nineteen, have never had diabetic ketoacidosis, and are taking less than 40 units of insulin per day you may have the adult-onset type of diabetes. If so a vigorous program of exercise and an HCF diet, under your doctor's close supervision, may help you to discontinue insulin therapy.

5. If you have juvenile-type diabetes, we can be much more optimistic now than we were five years ago. With home blood sugar measurements you can make much more intelligent decisions about your own insulin, diet and exercise program. If your diabetes requires an insulin infusion pump, these are now widely available. Many juvenile-diabetes are well controlled with insulin pumps after years of frustration and poor control using conventional insulin injections.

If you have diabetes mellitus of any type or category, the 1980s offer great hope. You can, with coaching from your doctor and health team, take charge of your diabetes. This will give you more control over your life, help you to make it fuller and healthier, and greatly reduce the likelihood of diabetic complications. I hope the information I have given in this book will help you cope better with living with your diabetes.

WHERE TO GET HELP

UNITED STATES

The American Diabetes Association
600 5th Avenue
New York, NY 10020

Juvenile Diabetes Foundation
23 East 26th Street
New York, NY 10010

National Diabetes Information Clearing House
NIH-NIAMDD
Room 628
Westwood Building
Bethesda, MD 20205

BRITAIN

The British Diabetic Association Ltd
10 Queen Anne Street
London W.1.
(Tel: (01) 323 1531)

CANADA

The Canadian Diabetes Association
123 Edward Street
Suite 601
Toronto
Ontario M5G 1ER
(Tel: 416 593 4311)
Contact: Marie Virgin, MD

AUSTRALIA

Doctors and other professionals in the field of diabetes should contact:
The Australian Diabetic Society
Secretary: Dr Alford
c/o Endocrine Unit
St Vincent's Hospital
Fitzroy
Victoria 3065

Members of the public should contact:
The Diabetic's Federation of Australia
5th Floor
Lombard Building
17 Queen Street
Melbourne
Victoria 3000

NEW ZEALAND

The New Zealand Diabetic Association
PO Box 3656
Wellington

WEIGHTS AND MEASURES

Both imperial and metric measures are given where appropriate. You may find the following simple conversions helpful:

30 g = 1 oz	30 ml = 1 fluid oz
15 g = $\frac{1}{2}$ oz	15 ml = $\frac{1}{2}$ fluid oz
10 g = $\frac{1}{3}$ oz	10 ml = $\frac{1}{3}$ fluid oz

American culinary measurements are cups and tablespoons.
An American measuring cup holds 8 fluid oz, and an American tablespoon holds $\frac{1}{2}$ fluid oz. When measuring solids as cups or tablespoons they are measured level.

British readers are recommended to work out the quantity of food equivalent to each exchange using their own cup or tablespoon as these vary in Britain.

Blood sugar measurements are expressed in this book as mg per 100 ml and, where appropriate, as mmol per liter. The latter system is part of the internationally recognized version of the metric system—*Système International* (abbreviated SI). The conversion factors are as follows: 1 mg per 100 ml = 0.056 mmol per liter; and 1 mmol per liter = 18 mg per 100 ml.

ACKNOWLEDGMENTS

I would like to thank my wife Gay for her patience and dedication in typing the manuscript. Mae McPhetridge, RN, whose compassion and dedication to the care of our patients with diabetes has set an example for all of us who work with her, developed some of the instructional material used in this book. Finally, I am grateful to Sue Slatterly, Beverly Sieling and Wendy Lin Chen, PhD, for their help.
J.W.A
Lexington, 1981

The publisher would like to thank the following individuals and organizations for their permission to reproduce photographs and illustrations: Action Mirabel (photo taken at Mirabel Airport, Montreal), page 59; Ames Division of Miles Laboratories Ltd, England, page 28 (top and center rows); Lisa Clark, page 28 (bottom right); Mick Duff, page 133; Dunlop Sports Co Ltd, England, page 32 (center); Becton Dickinson Consumer Products (a worldwide leader in diabetes care, Rochelle Park, New Jersey 07662, USA), pages 44 and 45; Hypoguard Ltd, England, page 28 (bottom left); Rob Matheson for the food photographs on page 32 and in chapter nine except page 133; Medic-Alert Foundation, London, page 70 (bottom); Miller Services, Toronto, page 77; NFB Photothèque, Canada, page 53; Novo Laboratories Ltd, England, pages 46 and 47; Martin Oudejans, page 54; Adrian Pope, pages 32 (top), 55 and 73; Christian Rosenbloom, page 145; Wellcome Foundation Ltd, England, page 48; Douglas Wilson, Washington, pages 57, 58 and 60; J.D. Wilson, Canada, page 56.
The diagrams were drawn by Barbara Leaning, except for page 81 by Cathy Slatter. Thanks are also due to Dr Pat Judd of Queen Elizabeth College, University of London, and Sister Sue Judd of St Thomas's Hospital, London, for their advice on British diabetic dietary and medical practice respectively; and finally to Anne Fairbairn for information on diabetic diets in Australia.

INDEX

155

legs, nerve damage, 81–2
Lente insulin, 31, 39, 73
lipoatrophy, 52

marriage, 74–5
medicines, influence on diabetes, 21
menus, 109–30
minerals, in diet, 87–8
motor nerves, damage to, 82
mumps, 10
muscles, nerve damage, 82
myoinisitol, 82

nerve damage, 81–2
neuropathies, 82
NPH insulin, 31, 39–40, 41–2, 49–50, 73

obesity, 16, 31–4, 52, 61–2, 84, 88, 93–6
oral hypoglycemic agents, 16, 61–3

pancreas, artificial, 144; failure, 10, 12, 14, 16; transplants, 144, 146–9
pituitary gland, 10
plasma glucose tests, 29
pneumonia, 16
pregnancy, 75
protamine-zinc insulin (PZI), 39
proteins, 79, 80, 86–7, 105, 108

restaurants, eating in, 64–5
retinal detachment, 80, 81

semilente insulin, 39
sensory nerves, damage to, 82
side-effects, antidiabetes pills, 63; insulin, 41, 42, 51–2
skin, allergic reactions, 51, 63; infections, 17–18
smoking, 24, 84
soluble insulin, 38, 41–2, 49–50,

71, 73
steroid hormones, 21
strokes, 24–5, 79, 84, 88, 90, 91
subcutaneous fat, changes in, 52, 76, 145, 146
sugar, emergency supplies, 41, 66, 70; see also blood sugar
sugar-hemoglobin test, 29
sulfonylureas, 61
sweeteners, artificial, 91–2
syringes, 49–51

teeth, extraction of, 72–3
thirst, increased, 15, 6, 17, 21
thyroid gland, 10
tolbutamide, 63
transplants, islets, 147, 148–9; pancreas, 144, 146–9
travel, 66–70
triglycerides, 90, 100–1

ultralente insulin, 39
urea, 79, 80
uremic poisoning, 79, 80
urine, increase in, 15, 16, 17, 21; kidney disease, 79; sugar in, 17, 20
urine tests, children, 77; keeping records, 69; ketones, 19–20, 75–6; sugar, 25–7, 29–30, 39–40, 68–9

veins, infusing insulin into, 146
virus infections, 10–11, 15, 75, 150
vision, blurred, 17, 74; see also eyes
vitamins, 87

weight loss, 15, 16, 17, 31–4, 52, 94–6

Other recently published health books:

DON'T FORGET FIBRE IN YOUR DIET
(American title: EAT RIGHT – TO STAY HEALTHY AND ENJOY LIFE MORE)

Denis Burkitt, MD, FRCS, FRS

This world-renowned medical scientist presents the first wide-ranging survey on the importance of fibre in preventing many typically western diseases.

BEAT HEART DISEASE!
Risteard Mulcahy, FRCPI, FRCP, MD

A reassuring look at one of today's most serious 'epidemics' – showing how changes in lifestyle could dramatically reduce the occurrence of heart disease and stroke.

OVERCOMING ARTHRITIS
Frank Dudley Hart, MD, FRCP

A leading rheumatologist describes just what arthritis and rheumatism are, and includes a wealth of ideas on how to keep your joints as supple and pain-free as possible.

ASTHMA AND HAY FEVER
Allan Knight, BSc, MD, CM, FRCP(C), FACP

Breathing difficulties or a streaming nose afflict thousands every year. Here an expert allergist explains what is happening to you and what you can do to ease the problems.

PSORIASIS
Ronald Marks, MB, BSc, FRCP, MRCPath

A leading dermatologist explains in simple terms everything you need to know about psoriasis, as well as how to cope with some of the practical and psychological problems it can present.

Forthcoming titles:
MIGRAINE AND HEADACHE
Marcia Wilkinson, DM, FRCP

HIGH BLOOD PRESSURE
Kevin O'Malley, MD, and Eoin T. O'Brien, MD